INSTRUCTOR'S MANUAL
TO ACCOMPANY

MOSBY'S

Fundamentals
of
THERAPEUTIC MASSAGE

Third Edition

SANDY FRITZ, MS

Founder, Owner, Director, and Head Instructor

Health Enrichment Center
School of Therapeutic Massage and Bodywork
Lapeer, Michigan

AMY HUSTED, AAS

Executive Assistant to Sandy Fritz

Lapeer, Michigan

with 29 illustrations

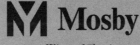
Mosby

An Affiliate of Elsevier

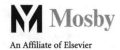
Mosby

An Affiliate of Elsevier

11830 Westline Industrial Drive
St. Louis, Missouri 63146

INSTRUCTOR'S MANUAL TO ACCOMPANY   ISBN 0-323-02684-2
MOSBY'S FUNDAMENTALS OF THERAPEUTIC MASSAGE

Copyright © 2004, Mosby, Inc. All rights reserved.

International Standard Book Number 0-323-02684-2

Publishing Director: Linda Duncan
Editor: Kellie Fitzpatrick
Developmental Editor: Jennifer Watrous
Publishing Services Manager: Linda McKinley
Senior Project Manager: Jennifer Furey
Cover Art: Julia Dummitt

GC/MVB

Printed in the United States of America

Last digit is the print number: 9 8 7 6 5 4 3 2 1

Contents

Introduction

The third edition of *Mosby's Fundamentals of Therapeutic Massage* is intended as a classroom and reference text. The textbook is designed to be used by skilled therapeutic massage educators in the classroom setting. This instructor's manual will help the instructor create a learning environment for the students.

The knowledge base in *Mosby's Fundamentals of Therapeutic Massage* has been increased to reflect the skills necessary for working effectively in the health care environment with supervision. Although my personal love for this profession lies in humble service to the general public in supporting wellness and compassion and help for the daily aches and pains of life, I also recognize the importance of working within the health care system. My work over the years with clinical physiologists and sport professionals supports this observation. Our task as instructors is to prepare the massage student for the current job market, and *Mosby's Fundamentals of Therapeutic Massage* will make this task easier.

HOW TO USE *MOSBY'S FUNDAMENTALS OF THERAPEUTIC MASSAGE*

The third edition has been extensively expanded to include knowledge that is necessary to function in diverse environments, such as general wellness practice, spa, sport, and medical massage. As with the last edition, the textbook has kept its effective work-text format. As the profession of therapeutic massage continues to become more sophisticated and the knowledge base expands, moving from recipe or routine approaches and applications to individualized therapeutic decisions becomes essential. Competency-based education requires integration of all curriculum information to be integrated into career skills. Instructors are faced more and more with the responsibility of teaching students to *think* in a professional manner and also develop the ability to record

this process in effective written records. More than ever, I am convinced that a strong understanding of the fundamental concepts of massage and the ability to effectively reason through a decision-making process are essential for a proficient professional practice. As instructors, we have the opportunity to teach in a way in which the student is able to eventually become his or her own teacher.

The decision-making process presented in the textbook is compiled from many systems and teaches a model of reasoning that can be used consistently when making different types of decisions. The model is as effective for ethical decision making as it is for charting decisions or for deciding what methods would be most effective to achieve a therapeutic goal, whether it be relaxation and a 1-hour vacation from life, enhanced athletic performance, symptomatic relief from years of chronic pain, or rehabilitation from an injury.

The challenge to instructors is to move beyond simply presenting the information and teaching the application of the modalities into acting as a guide as students manipulate that information in multiple ways while they learn to make effective decisions to achieve competency. The instructor will discover the importance of letting go of specific right and wrong answers and looking more for the student's ability to justify the effectiveness or appropriateness of the decisions being made. Throughout the text, the model for decision making will be used in activities, exercises, and case studies. Students will be challenged to sort and analyze the information and come up with their own decisions. *There are no single correct answers to these activities, exercises, and case studies any more than there is a correct way to do massage in the therapeutic setting.*

Competency-based learning and teaching requires that all information offered in a curriculum combines, overlaps, and supports professional skills in therapeutic massage practice. To support this success, the design of this instructor's manual contains suggestions for combining the information from both *Mosby's Fundamentals of Therapeutic Massage* and *Mosby's Essential Sciences for*

Therapeutic Massage: Anatomy, Physiology, Biomechanics, and Pathology, second edition, during instruction. *Mosby's Fundamentals of Therapeutic Massage* is a comprehensive skill-based text; but without the foundation of the sciences, the underlying mechanisms of the effects are confusing. Each textbook supports the other. If other textbooks are being used, this instructor's manual can assist in the integrated competency-based instruction that is necessary for the professional practice of therapeutic massage. Other educational material that should be incorporated into instruction, such as *Mosby's Fundamentals of Therapeutic Massage* Video Series and *Mosby's Massage Therapy Review with CD-ROM,* are also referenced in this instructor's manual. The EVOLVE site for instructors provides additional support.

Suggested Syllabus and Lesson Plan Guidelines for *Mosby's Fundamentals of Therapeutic Massage*

Introduction and Overview

Providing an overview of the text structure is important so the student becomes familiar with the design of the text. This objective can be accomplished by flipping though the text and identifying the basic components, including the interactive nature of the text, how the activities are laid out, and where the workbook sections and answer keys are located. This time is appropriate to discuss learning styles with the students.

CHAPTER 1: FOUNDATIONS OF THERAPEUTIC APPLICATIONS OF TOUCH (4 HOURS)

Chapter 1 begins with an exploration of touch and then describes the historical foundation of massage. The chapter provides the foundation on which our profession rests. The instructor's effective presentation of this material requires that students are able to explore their own values, history, and interpretation of touch interactions.

CHAPTER 2: PROFESSIONALISM AND LEGAL ISSUES (24 HOURS)

Chapter 2 introduces the clinical-reasoning/problem-solving model for ethical decision making. The focus is on making ethical decisions, but important to reinforce is that the model will be used for many different types of decisions. Principles of ethical behavior, communicated skills, and conflict management are presented.

CHAPTER 3: MEDICAL TERMINOLOGY FOR PROFESSIONAL RECORD KEEPING (12 HOURS)

Chapter 3 builds on Chapter 2 to include developing effective record-keeping skills. The first part of the chapter is devoted to terminology. This portion of the chapter is not meant to be an inclusive anatomy and physiology definitions course. The focus is on the way in which scientific (medical) terminology is used in written records. This chapter supports the instruction of anatomy and physiology. If the student is also using *Mosby's*

Essential Sciences as the anatomy and physiology textbook, Chapter 3 of both texts are similar and support each other.

The challenge in the instruction of Chapter 3 is that students are just beginning to develop history-taking and physical-assessment skills and do not yet have the technical skills or knowledge to combine the collected information with the application of massage. Reinforcement of the process will evolve throughout the course of study. If this information on charting and record keeping is not presented in the beginning and reinforced throughout the course of study, students have a tendency to discount the importance of these procedures, particularly record keeping.

CHAPTER 4: THE SCIENTIFIC ART OF THERAPEUTIC MASSAGE (8 HOURS)

Chapter 4 explains the research findings that support the benefits of massage. Based on the concept of *why massage works,* the chapter supports the concreteness of massage applications. The chapter also supports the anatomy and physiology instruction, providing relevance to the information presented in this portion of the student's studies. *Mosby's Essential Sciences* is recommended as the anatomy and physiology text because practical application of the anatomy and physiology is inherent in that text. If this book is not being used, the anatomy and physiology information will need to be made practical within the student's educational experience in terms of its functional relationship to massage applications.

CHAPTER 5: INDICATIONS AND CONTRAINDICATIONS FOR THERAPEUTIC MASSAGE (8 HOURS)

Chapter 5 begins the process of decision making in terms of indications and contraindications to massage. The decision-making process takes on a more practical application at this point. Case studies are used to support the clinical reasoning process.

CHAPTER 6: HYGIENE, SANITATION, AND SAFETY (4 HOURS)

Chapter 6 presents information regarding sanitation practices, standard precautions, personal health, and safety in the massage environment and preventing transmission of human immunodeficiency virus (HIV), hepatitis, and tuberculosis.

CHAPTER 7: BODY MECHANICS (24 HOURS)

Chapter 7 discusses massage equipment and the importance of proper use of the body while giving a massage. *Mosby's Fundamentals of Therapeutic Massage* Video Series can be used as an additional teaching source.

CHAPTER 8: PREPARATION FOR MASSAGE: EQUIPMENT, SUPPLIES, PROFESSIONAL ENVIRONMENT, POSITIONING, AND DRAPING (8 HOURS)

Chapter 8 builds on Chapter 7 and discusses draping procedures, various massage environments, supplies, and other information that is important to a successful massage practice. *Mosby's Fundamentals of Therapeutic Massage* can be used as an additional teaching source.

Chapter 9: Massage Manipulations and Techniques (64 hours)

Chapter 9 begins the technical skill chapters. Each chapter builds on the previous chapter, beginning with the basics, massage routines, and variations. Video support is available.

Chapter 10: Assessment Procedures and Care Plan Development (40 hours)

Chapter 10 teaches the student to perform an assessment and develop an individual care plan. With massage expanding more and more into the medical field, the massage practitioner's skills in this area are becoming more demanding. Gait and firing patterns have been expanded.

Chapter 11: Complementary Bodywork Systems (24 hours)

Chapter 11 expands therapeutic applications for specific populations, as well as an introduction to complementary bodywork systems and spa services. Sufficient information is presented in Chapter 11 to integrate simple methods from various bodywork systems other than therapeutic massage. Asian bodywork methods have been expanded. Respect for these systems acknowledges that each is a comprehensive study unto itself. Along with building an expanded knowledge base for the student, the instructor will also have the opportunity to reinforce the importance of respect for various complementary modalities, as well as to provide direction for continuing education.

Chapter 12: Serving Special Populations (24 hours)

Chapter 12 focuses on special populations, and the students should be able to see that the massage methods are fairly basic regardless of the situation or the environment; the people with whom we work are complex.

Chapter 13: Wellness Education (8 hours)

Chapter 13 explores general wellness education and fitness.

Chapter 14: Business Considerations for a Career in Therapeutic Massage (24 hours)

Chapter 14 discusses a career in massage. The information is not intended as a small business course. Although learning business structure is important in massage education, to reproduce a comprehensive chapter on business operations would be similar to writing a book within a book. Business is business, marketing is marketing, and many support texts are available to teach this general information. This chapter does present relevant information that is unique to the massage profession. Sufficient information is provided for the student to understand basic business concepts, status of employment, requirements for setting up a business, and self-reflection on what type of business structure within which the student wishes to work. Again, the chapter provides opportunity for the student to make decisions.

Chapter 15: Case Studies (24 hours)

Chapter 15 is a new chapter that contains 20 comprehensive case studies used to integrate the information from this text with science information to complete the competency-based outcome of education.

Massage Education and Competency-Based Instruction

Teaching therapeutic massage is unlike any other educational process. Students drawn to therapeutic massage are commonly interested in a model of education that mimics their expectations of the compassionate profession they have chosen to enter. Students seek technical information but also expect proactive application presented in a caring and integrated format.

Competency-Based Instruction

Competency-based instruction is focused on the mastery of skills that will be used as part of a professional practice. As instructors prepare lessons, they should ask themselves, "How will students actually use this information in the practice of therapeutic massage? What does this material have to do with therapeutic massage?" If instructors cannot logically and rationally answer these questions about the information they are presenting, they should consider eliminating it. Box I-1 on page viii presents guidelines to develop an educational program based on competencies.

Uniqueness of Therapeutic Massage Education

The concept of wholeness is pervasive in the massage and bodywork community. Students expect the education they receive to model this concept. The integrated nature of the education, the necessary awareness of self, the unique dynamics that concentrated instruction creates, and the practical exchange of touch in the classroom generates group dynamics that are not typically found in most classroom environments.

The student groups (classes) often begin to act as *families,* experiencing all the joys and frustrations found in this type of interaction. If the instructor takes on the role of *parent,* students are likely to act as *children.* Care needs to be taken to manage the group dynamics in such a way that the environment and educational approach remains warm, connected, compassionate, and yet professional, with appropriate boundaries among students, as well as between instructing staff and students. An adult educational model based on competencies, as described in this text, helps in managing these dynamics.

Also important to note is that a certain type of personality tends to be drawn to massage therapy education. Students with learning styles that take in information based on fundamental concepts and the *big picture,* as opposed to specifics and details, are a bit more common in the massage classroom. Many instructors seem to be concept oriented as well. This combination creates an effective educational structure for approximately 60% to

BOX I-1

Guidelines for a Competency-Based Education

Competency-based education will:

- Focus on student learning and performance, rather than on instruction, teaching techniques, textbooks, and instructor activity.
- Emphasize student mastery of skills, habits, and attitudes that represent actual job requirements and situations.
- Give students opportunities to solve problems and apply information and skills instead of simply answering questions about a topic.
- Require students to demonstrate knowledge and skills in ways that are observable by both the students and instructors.
- Shift the focus of the traditional classroom from teacher performance to student performance, from teaching to learning, from instructors presenting to students presenting, and from instructors teaching to instructors guiding students as they teach themselves.
- Present program content that is based on actual workplace application of the material being covered instead of a specific topic-by-topic approach. This approach requires an integrated education structure in which all material, science, theory, practical skill, ethics, communications, skills, and so forth are interrelated instead of being taught as separate ideas.
- Require the active involvement of students in the learning process instead of passive listening.

Competency-based lessons:

- Build on actual career expectations and applications.
- Include performance activities as early in the program as possible.
- Require students to think and perform like actual massage professionals.
- Provide students with opportunities to create, solve problems, and develop solutions based on justification instead of the "right answer."
- Teach students how to monitor and evaluate their own performance instead of relying only on instructor evaluations.
- Provide an opportunity for students to be active participants during classroom time.

- Minimize instructor lectures and maximize student study groups, small-group work in the classroom, individual or group presentations, and projects.
- Emphasize hands-on practical application of material instead of lecture and discussion.
- Provide performance objectives that are clear to students yet allow an opportunity for creativity, as long as students can appropriately justify their position.

Competency-based assessments:

- Measure students' performance against actual professional standards instead of against one another.
- Allow students the opportunity to ask intelligent questions to which responses are justified instead of maintaining the stance of the "correct answer."
- Require students to integrate all content into practical applications instead of only being able to perform a technique or routine.
- Test for the integrated understanding of course objectives instead of the simple ability to memorize a list of facts about the topics.

Strategies for teaching in a competency-based style include:

- Well-defined student outcomes for the entire program—not just individual classes
- Defined standards by which these outcomes will be measured
- Scenarios for role-playing, case studies, and problem-solving activities
- Guidelines for students to use in evaluating their own performance, including teaching students to provide objective feedback about their performance
- Development of an educational partnership with the student, redefining the role of the instructor from leader to coach, from being directive to being supportive, from an emphasis on delivery of information to reflection—with the end result being validation of the student's understanding

Adapted from Haron L: *Instructor's curriculum guide to accompany Gail A. Chester's modern medical assisting,* Philadelphia, 1999, WB Saunders.

70% of the students. However, the students who best learn when they are provided specific detail and linear structure may become frustrated with the educational delivery. In addition, constraints on time availability in the classroom can become frustrating for the students who need repetition before understanding. Fortunately, the textbooks can provide this structure—if it is effectively pointed out to students.

On the other hand, if the instructor uses a highly detailed, factually oriented approach to presenting infor-

mation, students who learn best by concept processing may get lost in the data. This style tends to happen in many science courses. Fortunately, *Mosby's Essential Sciences,* a companion text book to *Mosby's Fundamentals of Therapeutic Massage* offers big-picture, practical application that is relevant to the practice of therapeutic massage throughout the textbook.

Generally, people process information they receive in two ways. Some people process by framing information around human behavior, satisfaction, or meeting various human needs, such as social support, ego, and self-preservation. Other individuals process by focusing on practical implementation aspects, such as efficiency, practicality, cost, time, and the assumption that people will adjust themselves to what is most logical.

The therapeutic massage profession seems to attract people who are most influenced by feelings, emotions, and human interactions. Individuals who process by logic and cause and effect are rare in the profession. This tendency is unfortunate because these individuals bring a necessary and important balance to the classroom—and to the profession. Nonetheless, conflict may occur because people with a more logical processing style may challenge the practicality of certain information and question whether some activities are applicable to a professional practice. These individuals may seem a bit *cool* in regard to the human elements and not very open to the social interaction during class when the time comes to get down to the business of learning. Instructors of this style may seem distant or uncaring to the majority of students. Although this perception is biased, problems will occasionally occur in these group dynamics.

Regardless of learning style, information for this population of students needs to be practical and applicable to therapeutic massage. Material needs to be eliminated if it cannot be directly related in some way to the application of massage. The instructing staff develops the bridge from material to practical application. This process occasionally breaks down when instructors who are unfamiliar with massage teach the program. The two areas in which this breakdown most commonly occurs are the sciences and courses in business and professional application. For example, although fundamentals of ethics are fairly universal, applying ethical decision making to the practice of massage results in unique circumstances. An academic ethics professor who has never been in a massage room, either as a client or as a practitioner, will not have the experience to relate to these particular situations.

Therefore it is recommended that, regardless of the course component, each instructor should be familiar with therapeutic massage. The most effective instructor is also a massage-bodywork practitioner. Instructors who have received therapeutic massage and have read and studied *all* of the texts being used in the program—not simply those that focus on their particular area—can also be effective.

Student groups easily become enmeshed because of the close contact that ongoing interactions in massage therapy training generates. On the upside, this closeness results in cohesive supportive groups that help one another. On the downside—and just as common—is the breakdown of the group into factions: "us verses them." The diversity of learning and processing styles is often the underlining basis for this division. The student group may often line up against an instructor that does not *fit*

their collective ideal. Dissension can also manifest as small factions within groups. Also common is the *outcast student* who does not fit well with the rest of the group.

When any of these issues develops, the educational process is severely disrupted. Effective management of these situations can occur by discussing the potential of competency-based instruction, maintaining the adult learner educational partnership, and ongoing support for diversity. Both instructors and students benefit from an appreciation of diversity, learning how different people take in and process information in a decision-making process. An additional source for information on managing these issues, based on multiple educational resources and models, is the Myers-Briggs Type Indicator (MBTI). Many support materials are available for MBTI application in education and group understanding and dynamics. Other models are also viable. Further study in this area of group dynamics will greatly assist instructors in understanding human behavior.

Most massage and bodywork educators respond the same when asked about the dynamics of a therapeutic massage classroom. These educators will likely say that the dynamics of the classroom experience are significantly different from those found, for example, in computer schools. An understanding of this uniqueness needs to be inherent in the curriculum design to support successful outcomes.

The textbooks *Mosby's Fundamentals of Therapeutic Massage* and *Mosby's Essential Sciences* support a balance in these learning processes and encourage an appreciation and usage of all methods of learning—facts and details, intuition, possibilities and concepts, cause and effect—the pros and cons of each method based on factors of efficient process, including time, cost-effectiveness, ease of application, and compassionate understanding for the people involved.

Educational Environment

This instructor's manual is based on an integrated approach. If a program uses generalized classes that do not focus specifically on practical application integrated into therapeutic massage, some bridging classes will need to be offered—for example, Practical Application of Functional Anatomy and Physiology for Therapeutic Massage. Such a course would then allow students to learn about bones in true relation to how this information will be used during the application of massage. In this way, the general classes provide the individual pieces of the puzzle—bone, muscles, vessels, balance sheets, rental agreements, contracts, Swedish massage, shiatsu, muscle energy techniques, medical terminology, record keeping, charting, and so forth. Bridge classes take the pieces and put the puzzle together within the therapeutic massage framework.

Trends toward National Competencies and Standardization

The massage therapy profession is in an ongoing, active process of standardization. The number of state licensing examinations is increasing, and the National Certification Examination for Therapeutic Massage and Bodywork currently provides a competency-based, objectively designed tool to measure competencies. The challenge in the educational process is for educators to let go of their preconceived ideas, as well as any prior training and habits that fragment the educational process. Research shows that massage and bodywork methods interact similarly with physiology. Still common are curriculums designed around individual modalities, such as classes in Swedish massage, reflexology, deep-tissue massage, acupressure, stretching, sports massage, and prenatal massage, with each modality being presented as a separate entity instead of a piece of a whole. Instead of teaching specific modalities or applications, the responsibility of instructors is to guide students in developing an understanding of the fundamental applications of massage and bodywork methods so that they are able to make appropriate decisions about professional applications once they graduate and begin professional practice.

As the push toward standardization continues to influence therapeutic massage, applications will inevitably shift from modality (e.g., this is how you do effleurage) to gliding methods that are applied horizontally on the body and produce psychologic effects.

Competencies for the Professional Practice of Therapeutic Massage

In general, the competencies required for a successful practice of therapeutic massage fall into three areas:
- "Head" learning
- "Hand" learning
- "Heart" learning

Head learning involves the facts, concepts, and theories presented in the textbooks and current research in the field. This learning is important but is not completely adequate for practicing therapeutic massage.

Hand learning represents the applications of practical skill—giving massage. Hand, or kinesthetic, learning evolves from head learning. Understanding why (head) and without knowing how (hand) is insufficient; knowing how without the factual basis of why is inadequate as well.

Heart learning is the compassionate, professional respect for individuals that massage serves. Heart learning is the willingness to look deep within ourselves honestly and strive toward acceptance and respect for others and ourselves. A touch delivered from the heart is a skilled caring touch. Skilled touch (hand learning) without heart is empty.

The three Hs are essential in educating future massage practitioners as well. As instructors, we need to teach with our heads, hands, and heart. The three types of learning are presented in *Mosby's Fundamentals of Therapeutic Massage*.

The primary head knowledge chapters are Chapters 3, 4, 5, 14, and 15; the primary hand knowledge chapters include Chapters 6, 7, 8, 9, 10, and 11; and the primary heart knowledge chapters are Chapters 1, 2, 5, 8, 12, and 13.

Four Categories of Professional Therapeutic Massage Competencies

The information base that is required to function as a massage professional can be divided into four areas. These categories form the basis of most licensing and certifying examinations. The four categories are as follows:

1. Human Anatomy, Physiology, and Kinesiology

Program time allocated to this content section is generally 30% of the course. This general education prepares students to understand benefits of massage and lays the foundation for the following section.

2. Clinical Pathology and Recognition of Various Conditions and Indications and Contraindications for Massage Application

Program time allocated to this content section is generally 20% of the course.

Human anatomy, physiology, kinesiology, clinical pathology, and indications and contraindications for massage application cover one half of the available classroom hours. The focus is to provide sufficient information to support safe and beneficial professional practice.

This content is found in the textbook in Chapters 3, 4, 5, 12, 13, and 15.

Categories 1 and 2 are usually most effectively presented in an integrated format. For example, discussing the nervous system leads to an understanding of how massage affects the functions of the nervous system, which leads to understanding how massage affects nervous system, which leads to identification of indications for massage and the nervous system, which leads to pathology of the nervous system, which leads to contraindications for applications of massage, including cautions for use of massage when a pathologic condition is present.

Many people find the sciences a more difficult learning and teaching area. The terminology may seem overwhelming, similar to learning another language. If we can agree that the various methods and theoretical bases of the many different bodywork modalities provide diversity, then the sciences provide commonality. The human body in structure and function remains consistent; therefore, logically, an understanding of the sciences is essential—but it needs to be relevant to massage. In-depth discussion of the distribution of taste receptors on the tongue may be interesting; however, it is not often useful in massage application. Although students need to understand digestion, memorizing all of the specific digestive enzymes may appear as *overkill*. Knowing the name of every tooth and its specific function is important to a dental hygienist but not to a massage professional.

Mosby's Essential Sciences automatically sorts the anatomy and physiology content into information relevant for therapeutic massage. A generalized anatomy and physiology textbook does not. If you find using a standard anatomy and physiology text necessary, at least obtain a copy of *Mosby's Essential Sciences* to assist in sorting the content in the generalized anatomy and physiology textbook into relevancy to massage.

Non-Western science content is focused primarily on traditional Chinese medicine but also covers other energy systems such as shiatsu and Ayurveda. Chapter 11 of *Mosby's Fundamentals of Therapeutic Massage* covers this information sufficiently for an entry-level course.

Mosby's Essential Sciences integrates and correlates this information throughout the textbook.

3. Massage Therapy and Bodywork: Theory Assessment and Application

Competency in this area teaches the student to apply methods appropriately in a safe and beneficial way.

A commonality exists among most bodywork approaches. The content in this area covers various forms of assessment and interviewing methods to obtain essential information from the client. The information obtained from assessment then becomes the basis for applying safe and sanitary practices and enhances the appropriate choices of methods to be applied.

Approximately 40% of a course is allocated to this content, with approximately 15% of this category devoted to complementary bodywork modalities such as hydrotherapy, Asian theory, and applications such as acupressure, trigger points, and connective tissue massage.

Most of this content requires a hands-on application, thus lecture needs to be brief and concise. Make this area a practicum section with textbook support. Each of the listed chapters is set up as a *do* chapter. Many pictures and proficiency exercises are included to assist the practical teaching.

This content is found in the textbook as follows:
- Therapeutic massage theory: Chapters 4 and 5
- Assessment and treatment/care plan development: Chapters 3 and 10
- Technical skills—massage modality–based: Chapters 6, 7, 8, 9

- Theory and technical skills—complementary bodywork–based: Chapter 11
- Theory and technical skill—population-based: Chapters 12, 13 and 15

Mosby's Essential Sciences has Practical Application sections throughout that can be used as instructional or support and integration material in conjunction with *Mosby's Fundamentals of Therapeutic Massage*.

4. Professional Standards, Ethics, and Business Practices

Approximately 10% of the course is allocated to this area. Unfortunately, this length of time is usually insufficient. The professional standards, ethics, and business practice area develops professional abilities to interact with clients, peers, and other professionals. Included in this content are ethical behavior, interprofessional communication, basic business operational practices, record keeping for both business and client records, and an understanding of the scope of practice.

Instructors should focus on delivering enough general information so that students can make good professional decisions. If a student is going to encounter professional difficulties, they will likely stem from interpersonal dynamics and boundary issues and not that a name of a muscle is forgotten.

This content is found in the textbooks as follows:
- Technical skills—documentation, history taking, charting, client files: Chapters 3 and 15
- Professional skills—communications skills, interpersonal skills: Chapters 2, 9, 13, and 15
- Professional skills—ethics and ethical decision-making: Chapter 2
- Business and practice management: Chapter 14

The course is most effective when content is relevant to massage practice and students are taught how to find necessary information in the textbooks. Discourage memorization, but realize that both science and therapeutic massage have a language that must be learned to understand and communicate effectively. Students will need this language base to interact professionally. The key terms found in each chapter of both textbooks build the foundation for this language base. Students should be able to understand and use these terms correctly. Use the glossaries found in the textbooks to support learning of the key terms.

In addition, a professional expectation is that students should know the name, location, and function of the bones and bony landmarks, joints and associated structures, and muscles. The names of the major arteries, veins, nerves, and nerve plexus are also considered part of this language. If a term in the textbooks is boldfaced or italicized, students should be able to understand and use the term correctly.

Adult Learner—Developing the Educational Partnership

Students who are pursuing a therapeutic massage education become involved in postsecondary education. These individuals have chosen to be in school, and they have chosen to learn therapeutic massage.

At the beginning of the educational process, the instructing staff needs to set realistic expectations in an informed consent process so that students understand the extent of the learning that is required to practice massage professionally. Students are often surprised at the depth and breadth of the information and the proficiency that are necessary to practice massage professionally. Massage is a manual labor–intensive occupation. The labor intensity will be overwhelming if the student does not learn effective body mechanics. The effectiveness of body mechanics ensures that a therapist will be able to work an 8-hour day (six 1-hour sessions), without exhaustion and overexertion, 5 days per week. Students need to understand that a typical massage practice does not fit into a 9-to-5 schedule and that a typical workweek for a full-time practice can span 60 hours.

Students need realistic expectations about projected income. The national average is currently between $25,000 and $35,000 for full-time work (20 to 25 sessions over 40 to 60 hours per week). Although some professionals earn more, this level is the exception rather than the rule.

The amount of time required to achieve competencies is surprising. The financial considerations and obligations for the necessary education are important factors to consider. Schools should determine whether a student has a strong likelihood of completing the course of study successfully before accepting the student into the program. If students are not able to commit to the time required for study or do not have the financial stability to meet the cost of tuition, fees, and supplies, they should be informed that the likelihood of a successful outcome is poor. Each student should review the textbooks, meet with school representatives, and receive an orientation. This effort is all part of the informed consent process that supports an educational partnership between the school and the student.

Once the student has made an informed choice to enroll, the next stage of the educational partnership is determined. This aspect of the agreement emphasizes that the student has the responsibility for ensuring success in the program. Making students learn is not the responsibility of the instructing staff. Students are not passive in the educational process but instead are interactive participants. Competency-based instruction supports this process.

Adult learning is predicated on the premise that students will be self-motivated, responsible, and proactive in their learning. Therefore instructing staff members should not act as babysitters or truant officers. However, the instructing staff must be willing to be open to the evolution of the material as adult learners manipulate the information, blending it with other professional or life experiences. To achieve this objective, instructors will need to let go of absolute control of the classroom and unrealistic expectations that all answers must be known or that only certain answers are *right*. A partnership means working together as a team. For an instructor not to know the answer—and to ask students to look it up—is acceptable.

Educational partnerships mean commitment to get the job done—whatever it takes. This task requires multiple methods of instruction. Flexibility, along with the stability of structure, is necessary. Although instructors provide the perimeters and experience and maintain the educational environment, they need to be open to learning *from* students as well. The classroom is not a place for ego but rather a place to process information. Ideally, instructors should hope that each of their students will become more competent than they are. Power struggles are detrimental to learning. Adults need to solve problems so as to resolve conflict. Frequently, the challenge is remembering that we are *all* adult learners in the classroom—both instructors and students. An educational partnership supports this type of constructive interaction.

Challenges and Rewards of Clinicians as Instructors

In therapeutic massage schools and programs, an instructing staff composed primarily of massage practitioners is common. This situation has its advantages and disadvantages.

Advantages:
- Instructors possess actual practical experience.
- Instructors understand the realistic application of the textbook material.
- Instructors have the experience necessary to make the material *come alive.*
- Instructors have access to real-life examples from their client base.

Disadvantages:
- Instructors may neglect presenting educational material in a broad-based manner, focusing instead on personal style.
- Instructors may resist learning new procedures if these procedures are in conflict with their personal style.
- Instructors may have difficulty delivering information in a variety of methods that accommodate different learning styles.

The disadvantages can be minimized if clinicians are provided in-service training on instructional strategies, required to receive ongoing continuing education, and involved in peer support groups and supervision to share ideas, problem-solve difficulties, and benefit from experienced mentors.

Instructing staff members who do not have an understanding of massage application are often ineffective in the classroom. Some states or other regulatory bodies require that all science instructors have a degree. Many schools have responded by going outside the massage community for their instructing staff. This response can create difficulties when instructors with only academic experience and training in fields other than massage attempt to correlate scientific information with practical application for therapeutic massage. This same problem can occur with ethics courses; mental health professionals are often called upon to present this content. Although this choice may seem logical, these professionals do not typically touch clients, thus their practical experience is limited. Finding qualified instructing staff in these areas is difficult. A possible solution would be to team-teach these courses, with an instructor who is a massage professional providing the practical aspect.

Challenges and Rewards of Working with Multiple Instructors

In most educational programs, multiple instructors are responsible for various aspects of the curriculum. Using multiple instructors broadens educational experiences for students, allows for people with certain areas of expertise to focus on specific content, and provides variety in instructional style.

Of course, difficulties can arise if instructors operate independently of one another, especially when unified goals are necessary for competency-based education. All instructors must understand the criteria for successful student outcomes. Working together as a team will help achieve these objectives.

Teamwork and unified goals can be achieved through standardized instructional materials, master syllabus design (with each course having substitute instructors), and regular team meetings for curriculum development.

The most common separation occurs between the science instructing staff and the practical application instructing staff. These two groups of instructors need to coordinate and support each other instead of operating independently if a cohesive program is to be achieved.

Classroom Strategies and Educational Procedures

Various approaches and methods are used to present information to students. Lecture, demonstration, video, practicum, small groups, individual study, homework, independent study, student clinics, and externships are all methods commonly used.

Lecture
Lecture is the least effective method of presenting information for competency-based training. Lecture is a passive form of learning in which the student does not play an active role in the process. If an instructor chooses lecture as an educational strategy, he or she should expand or clarify information in the textbooks as opposed to simply restating information from the texts. When working with adult learners, instructors should expect that students have read or will read the textbooks. Also expected is that students are responsible for all information in the textbooks according to assignments. Lecture should present information not already found in the texts but based on the textbook readings. For example, credentials and licensing might be presented in lecture, describing the particular implementation of the process in the student's particular state or municipality. Description and elaboration of textbook information, based on the instructor's real-life experiences, provides excellent material for effective lectures.

If you choose lecture as an educational strategy, limit the time frame to a maximum of 30 minutes. Many students will be unable to maintain their attention on a subject after 30 minutes, even if the instructor is an effective lecturer. An effective lecture strategy is to choose a diagram or exercise from the textbook as a lecture focal point for each chapter or chapter section. Many of these figures are included as transparency masters in this instructor's manual.

The following are suggestions for lecture focal points from *Mosby's Fundamentals of Therapeutic Massage*:
- History—Figure 1-3 (historical time line)
- Scope of therapeutic massage practice—Figure 2-3
- Divisions of the nervous system—Figure 4-1
- Benefits of massage—Figure 5-1
- Relationship between the Five Elements and the organs—Figure 11-11

Involving the student in classroom discussion at various points within the lecture can support a more participating role for the student.

Video and Computer
Video presentations are a way to broaden the learning experience of the student. Using video presentations brings the expertise of other professionals to the classroom and expands on scientific information if using dissection videos or other media that assist in teaching the sciences. Make sure that any videos used in the classroom are approved for educational use, or obtain specific permission from the publisher. Mosby (Elsevier) has four videos that support the technical skills portion of *Mosby's Fundamentals of Therapeutic Massage*; support videos for anatomy and physiology instruction are also available. The Elsevier sales representatives will be pleased to provide information on these types of educational materials.

Treat video presentation as lecture. Break up the presentation through interaction with the video by starting and stopping it and encouraging class discussion.

Many web sites are available that support massage education on the Internet. Specifically, Elsevier offers the

EVOLVE site for both the student and instructor. For the instructor, this site has additional teaching information, links to study sites, a test bank, classroom materials, and so forth. For the student, the EVOLVE site is home to many activities throughout *Mosby's Fundamentals of Therapeutic Massage*. Each chapter contains an activity that directs the student online to his or her personal EVOLVE site where chapter concepts are enhanced through online activities.

Enclosed with this instructor's manual is a CD-ROM containing the information in this book in a downloadable format, enabling the instructor to build customized lesson plans, write examinations, and display transparencies in class.

Demonstration

Demonstrations are effective teaching strategies if students are able to practice the information immediately after seeing the demonstration (practicum). Demonstrating a complete massage for students at the beginning of the course is helpful so that they have a big-picture frame of reference—and have an idea of where the program is going. At this early point, the demonstration is not expected to be replicated.

Demonstration usually involves a portion of a process or methodology that is demonstrated, after which students replicate what they observed during the demonstration. Under most circumstances, demonstrations should be limited to 15 minutes, with adequate time provided for students to practice the demonstrated material.

All of the illustrations in Chapters 7, 8, 9, 10, 11, and 12 are appropriate and are included as an image bank on both the CD-ROM in this book and on the accompanying instructor's EVOLVE site.

Practicum

Practicum goes hand in hand with demonstration. Hands-on practice is the most effective way to instruct an adult competency-based program. A massage-training practicum involves using equipment, methods of draping, body mechanics, application of various massage manipulations and techniques, methods of assessment, intake and charting procedures, and so forth.

Grouping of various types can be used to support hands-on practice. Dyads (two students) can be formed with one student acting as the *body* and the other as the *practitioner*. Triads (groups of three) can also be effective. In this case, one student is the *body*, the second student is the *practitioner*, and the third student can play the role of tableside teacher or observer. The observer can then provide feedback while the other two students share the client and practitioner roles, teaching one another. Roles are reversed or rotated so that students experience all roles during the practical experience.

The dyad pattern takes less time in the classroom, but the opportunity for objective observation and feedback is minimal. The student acting as the *body* or *client* can

provide some feedback—but not as effectively as a third person with a designated observation role. Without an observer, the instructor has the sole responsibility of providing the observation and feedback.

The triad is highly effective because three students share information and feedback. Given that these individuals are responsible adult students, they are expected to provide appropriate, objective, accurate feedback to one another. Although this situation is uncomfortable at first for some students, the ability to learn and the opportunity to give and receive effective feedback is valuable. The triad supports the adult competency-based learning experience effectively. With this model, the instructor is able to move from group to group, accessing more students each time he or she acts as tableside teacher. The responsibility for objective feedback is shared between students and the instructor, again supporting the educational partnership.

Time frames for practicum vary. Care needs to be taken to provide sufficient time for students to practice without being rushed; at the same time, the instructor needs to watch for signals that indicate whether students are on task. If not monitored, students often become distracted from their objectives and valuable time is lost in the classroom. Typically, a 15-minute demonstration will require 30 minutes of practice time per student.

Small-Group Discussion and Presentation

Small-group discussion is a valuable instructor strategy. Small-group discussion can often replace a portion of a typical lecture. Combining discussion with presentations provided by small groups can eliminate most lecture in the classroom. Small groups of four to eight students are most effective; having an odd or even number of people in the groups is not typically important.

Various topics can be assigned to small groups so that students can work together to sort the information. Having students collaborate on case studies, problem-solving activities, or proficiency exercises found in both textbooks creates an effective dynamic in the classroom.

If students develop the information generated in group discussion into a classroom presentation, each member of the group must be an active participant instead of a passive participant. The responsibility of the instructor is to support the activity of the small groups, encourage participation, monitor the presentations for accuracy, and contribute additional information regarding the presentation.

For example, instead of the instructor lecturing and demonstrating information about various muscles, divide the classroom into small groups and assign each group a muscle or related group of muscles (such as the muscles of the rotator cuff). Instruct the groups to discuss the location, function, and relevant factors of each muscle. Have the groups prepare a presentation about their muscles and present it to the entire class.

Time frames vary, but 30 to 45 minutes of group discussion is usually adequate. Each group presentation should take between 10 and 15 minutes. Provide time for full-class discussion and feedback about the small-group presentation. This point is the time when the instructor can add or expand information or correct misinformation—if correction was not given while the group was presenting. This process can take 10 to 15 minutes. During the group presentations and discussions, the instructor is able to assess students' understanding of the information, which can often be a more accurate representation of students' knowledge than more formal testing procedures.

Individual Study, Presentation, and Research Papers or Projects

Another strategy is focused on individual study and presentation and supports students who prefer to work alone, as well as challenging each student to become his or her own teacher. Students should be given this option for at least a portion of the course. Being involved in some sort of individual study and providing a presentation for the rest of the class is beneficial for all students.

Specific syllabus topics can be assigned to individual students for development into classroom presentations.

Individual study often takes the form of a research paper or project. Students' topics should be proposed to the instructor for assessing their relevance in relationship to the course of study. For example, how to build a massage table would be relevant, whereas how to build a picnic table would not.

Independent Study

Independent study can be designed as either an individual or group activity. The focus of independent study is to encourage the students to reach for knowledge outside the textbook, but based on the foundation of information presented in the textbook. Many of the proficiency exercises in *Mosby's Fundamentals for Therapeutic Massage* offer suggestions that would be appropriate for independent study as well.

Essentially, students become their own teachers when involved in independent study. This educational strategy is appropriate to use in competency-based education once the fundamental information and skills have been presented.

Homework

Homework prepares students for participation in class activities and information integration. Homework consists of reading assignments and completing activities, exercises, and workbook sections in the textbooks. Homework can also consist of practical-skill practice outside the classroom. A common strategy in massage training is to require that each student complete a certain number of massage sessions or hours of practical-

massage practice outside of class. Students should log, chart, or journal the practice experience. These practice experiences can become a basis of class discussion or small-group interaction if the experiences are shared in a student group setting monitored by the instructor.

Understanding the nature of homework is important. Typically, students do not enjoy homework assignments. Therefore, a degree of flexibility is helpful. Some students will actually understand reading assignments better after the classroom presentation. These students usually do not consistently read assignments ahead of class. This aspect can become a point of conflict between student and teacher. A helpful compromise is to suggest that these students read the key terms and the answer keys in the workbook sections of the textbooks before the classroom presentations. Essentially, the answer keys provide chapter summaries. Although some instructors resist this idea, remember, we are teaching adult students—not children. The goal is to learn—however it happens. Offering options in homework is helpful. Instead of requiring everyone to do the same assignment, either provide two or more ways to complete the homework or have students tell *you* how they intend to accomplish the learning objective. Remember, the goal of homework is to prepare students for classroom learning, as well as to integrate the material presented. Encourage study groups so that students can work on homework together.

Student Clinics

Many programs incorporate some sort of practical experience in a student clinic setting. Student clinics give students the opportunity to practice their professional and technical skills with the public while under supervision.

Student clinics can be structured in many different ways. The classroom can be set up as a mock clinic with individuals from the community accessing students for massage. Arrangements can be made for students to go to various settings outside the classroom and provide massage. Potential settings include senior citizen centers, corporate offices, and local sporting events. This type of experience should not be considered an externship because the experiences are planned and supervised by school instructing staff. During clinical experience, the instructing staff should monitor students. Tableside teaching should occur, and the process should be developed as an interactive learning experience among the practice clients, student practitioners, and the instructing staff. Too often, the clinical experience becomes a time when students provide massage to the clinical patrons without direct interactive teaching from instructors.

A more beneficial learning process occurs when each practice client understands that students are involved in an active learning experience and that constructive feedback is important for students to continue to integrate and improve their skills. The practice client should be informed that instructing staff will be interacting with the student during the massage sessions, providing correction, suggestion, and reinforcement. Given the appropriate informed consent process, practice clients are usually open to this type of experience. If a potential client is not open to this environment, he or she should not be participating in student clinics.

Emphasis must be made to students that they are not yet involved in giving massage as professionals but are still learning. As such, students need to be open to feedback, to learning through tableside instruction, to accepting correction without becoming embarrassed or defiant, and to engage the client in an active learning experience.

Externships

Externships are designed for students to work in an actual professional environment. When externships are used as part of the educational process, the experience is usually scheduled toward the end of the program as part of a completion phase. Typically, a 100- to 150-hour sequence is necessary to best serve both the student and the externship site. An actual work schedule is expected and should be documented. The student is expected to integrate into the work environment as if he or she were fully employed in the job setting.

Externships are not necessarily supervised directly by instructing staff. Instead, an on-site supervisor is usually responsible for monitoring the progress of the student.

Typically, an externship agreement exists between the school and various work environments acting as extern sites. An attorney should be involved in the development of externship agreements to address liability issues. The agreement between the school and the work site agreement should include the following:

- Length of the agreement and method of termination
- Responsibilities of the school—for example, providing prepared students, evaluation criteria, the final grade assignment, assistance with student problems, and liability insurance for students
- Responsibilities of the externship site—for example, providing actual work opportunities and supervision, completing student evaluations, informing the school of student problems, and participating in corrective action if necessary

Students should receive an orientation for the externship experience from the school before being placed. All details of the experience need to be explained to the student, and a checklist of approved techniques to be used in the work setting should be provided.

Students should report to a school representative during an externship so that the educational process can be monitored.

Externships are not common in 500-hour programs; simply stated, not enough time exists. If, however, the program is longer than 500 hours, an externship can be a valuable educational component to the student's competency-based training.

Distance Learning

Although distance learning using current computer technology is not usually addressed in therapeutic massage education, this format of education is quickly becoming viable. Because distance learning is another form of independent learning, the participating student essentially becomes his or her own teacher. Appropriate instructional materials would be required to support this process.

The kinesthetic nature of therapeutic massage will always require a direct student-to-instructor interaction for the technical skills and integration of application to be taught effectively. However, a combined program using distance learning and residency classroom instruction might be a reasonable approach. Expecting that an entire therapeutic massage course might be presented in this format is unreasonable; thus extensive residency programs will continue to be a part of therapeutic massage education. Ignoring the possibilities of integrating a distance-learning component to therapeutic massage education is equally unreasonable.

Distance learning is not for all students. This type of learning requires self-motivation, discipline, and the ability to act as one's own teacher. However, the technology has evolved to allow more interaction with the instructor and fellow classmates and therefore is a vast improvement over the previous concept of *correspondence education*. By using online educational software, various interactions between the student and the instructor can take place. Chat rooms and other formats can also be used to support communication among students.

Because of these improvements, distance learning can be a valuable option for some students to fulfill part of their training requirements. Considering the concepts of *head, hand,* and *heart* learning, a reasonable assumption is that distance learning might be used to address much of the *head* learning of a curriculum. For instance, a large percentage of the sciences can be taught in a distance-learning format. Using a text such as *Mosby's Essential Sciences* is important because it is an interactive work text and bridges the sciences with the practical application within the text content. Of course, certain adjustments would need to be made. For example, Chapter 10 (Biomechanics) would not lend itself to distance learning, but the theory base of this chapter might be included. A reasonable assumption is that some sort of practical application course in residency format would have to be included to ensure that the student's understanding of palpation, movement, and other practical application was meeting required competencies.

Testing Procedures—Examinations

Written Examinations

The main purpose of any test is to measure competency in a particular area. Written examinations are usually used to measure competency in the sciences, massage theory, clinical reasoning skills, and professional skills such as charting. Two main types of written examinations are used: the essay examination and the multiple-choice examination. A combination of essay and multiple-choice questions is a common form of written examination design.

Essay Examinations

Essay examinations require students to respond to a question and then justify their response. Essay examinations seem best to measure students' competency in a particular subject. However, essay examinations are subjective and difficult to grade given that the instructor is often faced with responses to questions that may not agree with his or her interpretation of the correct answer. At times, no correct answer exists. Instead, the instructor looks for certain elements to appear in the response to the question and evaluates the skill with which the student answers the question. Additionally, the instructor assesses how well the student manipulates the information to demonstrate an understanding of the information presented.

Essay examinations may appropriately be open-book processes, allowing students to use various resources to formulate their responses. The responses to the questions should be based on the student's ability to manipulate the textbook information to support a meaningful answer. Memorization is not the goal.

The following is an example of a science-based essay question of this type: *Describe the feedback loop interaction between the sympathetic and parasympathetic proportions of the autonomic nervous system in relationship to the three stages of the general adaptation syndrome as described by Hans Selye.*

As you can see, students would need to understand a feedback loop, the homeostatic control functions of the autonomic nervous system, and the general adaptation syndrome—and be able to manipulate this information to explain the interaction of autonomic regulation and the stress response. Students can answer this question in many ways; they can write a narrative, develop a diagram, and provide examples.

The following is an example of a technique-based essay question: *Explain the differences and similarities between massage manipulations such as gliding strokes, compression, kneading, shaking, rocking, vibration, tapotement, friction, massage techniques using joint movement and various forms of muscle energy techniques, and stretching in relation to increasing arterial circulation to the limbs.*

Students would need to be able to understand how arterial circulation functions and how various massage methods increase arteriole circulation. Students would need to identify which massage manipulations and massage techniques are the best for increasing arterial circulation and then compare and contrast the various approaches. Again, students can approach an effective answer to this question in many different ways.

Most of the chapter objectives can be restated as essay questions. For example, in *Mosby's Fundamentals of Therapeutic Massage*, a Chapter 5 objective reads: *Define therapeutic change, condition management, and palliative care.* This objective can be reworded as an essay question: *Explain how decisions are made concerning when each of the following approaches would be appropriate to client care: therapeutic change, condition management, and palliative care.*

One of the objectives of Chapter 9 in *Mosby's Fundamentals of Therapeutic Massage* reads: P*erform a full-body massage using the methods and techniques presented.* Reworded as an essay question: *Design and describe in detail a 45-minute full-body massage session. Incorporate both massage methods and techniques. Describe each method chosen, justify your rational for the methods selected, and describe the expected results for the client receiving the massage, including explanation as to why they would experience the benefits described.*

Multiple-Choice Examinations

The multiple-choice examination is the most common examination process; it is easy to grade, has a defined correct answer for each question, and is more objective than the essay examination. However, the strengths of the multiple-choice examination are also its weaknesses. Although multiple-choice questions can be worded to require the student to use clinical reasoning, this is not commonly done in the typical multiple-choice examination. Instead, most multiple-choice examinations are written to elicit regurgitation of factual data. In this case, actual competencies are not likely to be measured effectively. Therefore if multiple-choice examinations are used, the questions must be carefully written. Multiple-choice questions are of three basic types:

1. FACTUAL RECALL AND COMPREHENSION

The information necessary to answer these questions can be found in the textbooks in the form of descriptions and definitions. Students can use memorization of data to prepare to answer these questions. Of the three basic types of questions, factual recall and comprehension questions are the easiest to develop and the most concrete in terms of right or wrong answers.

The following is an example of a factual recall and comprehension question:

Which bone makes up the heel of the foot?
a. Navicular
b. Calcaneus
c. Hamate
d. Xyphoid
The answer is b.

Labeling is another form of measuring students' factual knowledge. This approach is especially useful in anatomy examinations. The instructor's manual for *Mosby's Essential Sciences* contains masters for labeling examinations. An answer key is also provided.

2. APPLICATION AND CONCEPT IDENTIFICATION

This type of question requires that students understand the language posed in the question or be able to identify simple concepts and patterns. In addition, application and concept identification questions measure students' ability to understand language as it relates to contextual frameworks.

These questions also address concrete information that can be described in terms, definitions, rules, laws, and other forms of structure. This information can be found directly in the textbook base.

The following is an example of an application and concept identification question:

Which method would be most appropriate if the client desires to remain passive during the massage?
   a. Pulsed muscle energy
   b. Reciprocal inhibition
   c. Approximation
   d. Postisometric relaxation
The answer is c.

3. CLINICAL REASONING/SYNTHESES

Clinical reasoning/syntheses questions require students to manipulate information, analyze it, and make appropriate decisions. Identifying the answer to this type of question requires that the information be used in a contextual manner. Although these questions are more difficult to write, they are the most valuable in terms of measuring competencies. The case study scenario is a common approach to this type of question.

Answers to clinical reasoning/synthesis questions are not found directly in any textbook. Only the language and concepts necessary to answer these questions are in the textbooks.

The following is an example of a clinical reasoning-synthesis question:

Mrs. H. is taking aspirin for osteoarthritis of the left knee. What cautions are indicated for massage intervention?
   a. Avoid any type of massage to the affected knee.
   b. Avoid using compression above and below the knee.
   c. Reduce pressure level around the knee only.
   d. Monitor pressure levels of the massage to reduce potential bruising.
The answer is d.

The multiple-choice test banks in this text are based on factual recall and comprehension questions with a few clinical reasoning multiple-choice questions. Any of the case studies found in *Mosby's Fundamentals of Therapeutic Massage* can be a basis for developing this type of question. Problem-solving exercises in both textbooks also provide a basis for developing these questions. The text *Mosby's Massage Therapy Review* has over 800 multiple-choice questions for review. A sampling of these questions is located on the instructor's EVOLVE site to accompany this textbook.

The most difficult part of writing multiple-choice questions is developing plausible wrong answers. If the correct answer is too apparent, the student's competency is not measured. If the correct answer is not justifiable, or if an incorrect answer is actually a plausible solution to the problem posed by the question, the question is ambiguous.

Student-Written Examinations

An alternative examination development strategy—one that functions as a hands-on learning experience for students—is to have students write essay questions or multiple-choice questions as part of small-group work or individual study. In this approach, the student would write essay questions (with the intended answers), or multiple-choice questions of all three types, or both, indicating the correct answer from the four choices offered. If students can write effective examination questions and present justifiable answers, they are displaying competency for the area of study. Develop an examination question bank by collecting the best questions written by the students.

Testing Procedures—Practical Application

Practical examinations measure competency in technical skills. These tests are not as objective as are written examinations. Competence depends on students performing skills to the satisfaction of the instructor testing them. Some educators suggest that students be required to *explain* what they are doing as they demonstrate each technical skill. Instructors may be better able to understand students' intentions if they consider both what they observe and what students tell them as justification.

The usual procedure for practical examinations is that the student demonstrates proficiency in a technical skill area while being observed by an instructor. In massage programs, some instructors require that students perform the massage applications on the instructor to *feel*, as well as observe, how the student is doing.

Peer evaluation is a viable option for practical examinations. For this activity, students are divided into groups of three. One student is the practitioner, a second student is the observer, and the third student acts as the client. The responsibility of the students playing the client and the observer is to assess the competency of the student performing the massage or other technical skill, such as history taking or physical assessment.

This information is recorded on a feedback form and after the session is presented to the student who is being evaluated. This student then completes a self-evaluation form, giving himself or herself a grade, justifying the position and providing recommendations for self-improvement. All three students then present their information to the instructor for acceptance.

Each student plays all three roles during the practical examination process. This approach to examinations supports competency-based learning. During this type of examination procedure, students incorporate interactive learning from one another, develop observation and feedback skills, and learn to self-evaluate objectively. The process is validated because the instructor observes all peer evaluation groups and approves all self-evaluations.

Regardless of how practical examinations are constructed, students need to know by what criteria they are being measured. The Rubric competency document (see Appendix in the back of this manual) provides suggestions. Expectations should be established in a practical examination evaluation form. Figure App-1 before the Rubric in the Appendix is included as a model to be modified as needed.

Preparing Students for Examinations

Many students have had negative experiences with examination procedures. This circumstance creates the potential for test anxiety and even phobic behavior. Obviously, instructors will not be able to measure students' abilities accurately if the students are test-phobic.

To reduce test anxiety, allow students to see examinations before taking them and provide specific study guides. Conducting practice examinations to prepare students for the *real* test is helpful. Even choosing each student's best performance, whether on the practice examination or the real examination, can be helpful. Some students will perform better if they think they are taking a practice examination because their anxiety is lowered. Other students energize and perform best under pressure.

Instructors best serve students by being creative with examination procedures. In competency-based instruction, the outcome needs to reflect how the graduate will perform on the job. As long as you can measure this level effectively, allow yourself to be creative. Not all students can be evaluated by the same method. Provide flexibility.

Sort the information on your examinations carefully. If students will not use a particular piece of information on the job, or if they are not likely to encounter it on a certification or licensing examination, do not include it in your examinations, whether written or practical.

Memorization can begin the study process, but students must also develop an understanding of the context of the information. Do not require memorization of information that is better presented in a research approach that can allow students to look up data as needed. An example of this method is information about medication types or pathologic conditions. In the actual workforce, people use references. The ability to ask intelligent questions, use appropriate references, gather information, and analyze data for effective decision making is much more important than being able to name all the cranial nerves or digestive enzymes. In actual experience, a broader information base is used in decision-making applications. Students can begin to study by reviewing the content in the textbooks; however, memorization does not reflect understanding. Competency-based education is based on understanding (see Rubric and "Practical Examination Performance Evaluation").

LEARNING STYLES

Human behavior has recognizable patterns—sometimes called personality *style* or *temperament*—that have been identified as four basic methods of operating in the world. (See Types of Learners, later in the Introduction.) Although temperament is culturally and environmentally influenced, it seems to be genetic. Because each of us is a unique being, the manifestation of an individual's temperament is the sum total of all the person's experiences—applied to the initial imprint or basic underlying structure, which remains recognizable.

Style or *temperament* in education has particular relevance. When working with groups of people, structuring the educational delivery and environment to each individual in the class would be ideal. This ideal is not realistic; however, knowing a person's temperament does enable the instructor to understand and predict behavior and therefore attempt to vary classroom interaction to the four different temperament styles as defined in this Introduction. Thus the basic needs of all class members can be satisfied, and individualization can take place as needed on a one-to-one basis.

Teachers typically present in their preferred style and expect others to respond or understand. However, as an instructor, he or she must move beyond a person's individual preferred style and vary the instructional strategies to meet the needs of the class members. The further away from the teacher's preference a student's instructional style is, the more practice and understanding it takes for the teacher to recognize and appreciate that style. *Mosby's Fundamentals of Therapeutic Massage* considers different learning styles, both in the way it is written and in the design of the activity and workbook components.

In addition to the temperament styles of students, external forces exist in the classroom environment that have a direct effect on students. In essence, these forces are instructional strategies, curriculum content, and classroom atmosphere.

Instructional Strategies

Instructional strategies are the methods, tactics, or modes of instruction that a teacher uses to bring about a specific learning outcome. These strategies include discussions, demonstrations and lectures, assignments, games, and exercises. Teachers must know what tactics are most effective with each type of learner. *Mosby's Fundamentals of Therapeutic Massage* presents the textbook information in multiple ways so that the instructor may choose from a variety of instructional strategies.

Curriculum Content

Knowing the type of curriculum content that each style of learner prefers is an important ingredient for designing an effective educational program. Certain students will show a preference for science, and others will be more inclined to business, clinical, or interpersonal information.

Classroom Atmosphere

The classroom atmosphere is the impression that the environment creates in students. The classroom may have a friendly, warm, and personal atmosphere. The classroom may be one of working, playfulness, or discovery, or it may have an atmosphere in which students are cooperative and act as a cohesive group, or the atmosphere may be hostile, defiant, and stifled.

Some students may do best in a learning environment filled with spontaneity, fun, and excitement; others may need a friendly, secure, ordered atmosphere; still others may need harmony and democracy. The key to creating a variety of classroom climates evolves as the teacher's relationships with the students grow. To support the instructor in building these relationships, *Mosby's Fundamentals of Therapeutic Massage* presents a conversational, friendly tone while providing a structured approach to unfolding the content.

When the teacher begins to understand each student as having a certain type of personality and a particular learning pattern, he or she will no longer expect all students to be responsive to the same educational approach. Once a student's learning pattern is identified, the teacher can group students according to their similar learning patterns and teach students within each group using the same instructional methods and materials. Thus, rather than having one instructional program for all students, or a separate instructional program for each student, the educator who uses the methods in this instructor's manual and Mosby's therapeutic massage textbook line will be able to design a program to match each of the four learning (temperament) styles by offering multiple explanations of the same content and diverse activities and exercise patterns.

No one way is correct—all styles and temperaments are acceptable. Strengths are displayed by certain temperament styles, predisposing an individual to a preferred way of being and operating. The mix of diversity—all of the temperaments working together—can develop the most creative ideas and solutions to problems.

HOW PEOPLE PROCESS INFORMATION

When functioning in the world, we first take in the situation, think about it, react emotionally to the thoughts, and ultimately act on it. If the situation occurs often enough or is experienced with great emotional intensity, a conditioned response can occur. When we become conditioned (classic and operant conditioning, as described by Pavlov and Skinner) to a sequence of events, the *think about it* step is often bypassed on a conscious level, and we move directly to the reaction phase influencing behavior. One effect of conditioning is that even when we attempt to communicate differently as instructors, we find ourselves falling into the most familiar conditioned patterns, especially when stressed. Being able to recognize, consider, and accommodate various learning styles is important when attempting to relate to people whose temperaments differ from our own. This task is much easier said than done because conditioned habits make this adaptation process difficult.

- People perceive and gain knowledge, called *cognition.*
- People form ideas and think, called *conceptualization.*
- People feel and form values, called *affect.*
- People act, called *behavior.*

All of these actions are done differently by different people.

Cognition: "How Do I Know?"

Some of us perceive best what is real, whereas others see clear possibilities with their imaginations. Some people see the parts of a whole, separating the ideas from their context, whereas others see the whole (i.e., they see the trees or the forest).

Gaining knowledge is a part of cognition. People get information in different ways. Some people use abstract sources, reading about things and listening to the descriptions of others. Other individuals need concrete experiences. The *concrete person* often depends directly on the senses for information, needing to see it, do it, or feel it to know that it is true. The *abstract person* is more receptive to secondhand sources of knowledge. This type can imagine a vivid reality without needing to experience it. Sensory specialization, relying on the audio, visual, or kinesthetic sensory pathways, is a primary way of gathering and delivering information. *Mosby's Fundamentals of Therapeutic Massage* supports teaching and learning styles by using both concrete and abstract presentations. When the more concrete student attempts the more abstract activities, frustration or a lack of understanding can develop. Supporting such students will help them to develop their more abstract processing abilities. The more abstract learner, on the other hand, can find the concrete activities and presentations boring or dull.

These students will have the opportunity to practice the necessary discipline for many of the tasks of professional practice.

Conceptualization: "How Do I Think?"

People exhibit differences in what they do with the information they receive. Some people are convergers, always looking for connections and ways to tie things together. Other people are more divergent—one thought, idea, or fact triggers a multitude of new directions. Some people order ideas, information, and experiences in a linear, sequential way, whereas others organize their thoughts in clusters and random patterns. Some people think out loud; they verbalize ideas as a way of understanding them. Other people concentrate on understanding concepts and experiences privately in their own mind. Some people think quickly, spontaneously, and impulsively; others are slower, more reflective, and deliberate.

Affect: "How Do I Decide?"

Differences in motivation, judgments, values, and emotional responses also characterize individual style. Some people are motivated internally, and others seek external rewards and motivation. Some people actively seek to please others, and some are not attuned to the expectations of others. Still other people will rebel against such demands. Some people make decisions logically, rationally, objectively, and with cool heads. Some people decide things subjectively, focusing on perceptions and emotions, their own and others. Some people need frequent feedback on their ideas and work, whereas others are discouraged by the slightest criticism. Some people welcome analytical comments, and still others do not even ask an outsider for a critique.

Some people are emotionally involved in everything they do, and others are characteristically neutral. The emotional learner prefers a classroom with a high emotional charge, whereas the more analytic learner works best in a low-key, less emotionally charged environment. In other words, a balance of both is desired.

Behavior: "How Do I Act?"

Behavior is a direct action display of all the factors involved in the temperament of an individual. The reflective thinker can be expected to act in a reflective way. The spontaneous thinker will approach a task randomly, whereas concrete thinkers are systematic. Some people need explicit structure, and others prefer and perform best in a more open-ended situation. Some people prefer to work alone, and others do best in groups.

People who require structure and planning do best using schedules and lists, whereas others respond in the moment or wait until the last minute to respond or decide with what may seem as little planning at all.

TYPES OF LEARNERS

The four basic types (temperament) of learners are:
- Actual-spontaneous learner (ASL)
- Actual-routine learner (ARL)
- Conceptual-specific learner (CSL)
- Conceptual-global learner (CGL)

Actual-Spontaneous Learner (38% of Students)

For people who display this temperament, life is a process of making instantaneous decisions among an array of options. Born with a predisposition for keen observation of the specific and concrete in the present moment, these individuals tend to focus on the immediate and to be captured by whatever is happening and do whatever is expedient. Dull routine and structure put these people to sleep; perceived boredom is stressful.

These individuals are stressed by wordiness, abstraction, uneventful routine, restraint, and lock-step procedures.

The ASL prefers to learn from experience and considers it to be the best teacher. This group will appreciate the practical application sections in the textbooks and classroom.

As class work becomes more focused on study and preparation, these types of learners become uninterested. As the demand for concentration increases and activity decreases, these people become bored, restless, and not as attentive; they thrive on situations in which the outcome is unknown; they appreciate activities that have no specific correct answer and usually enjoy the puzzle of figuring it out; and they must do something if they are going to learn, and the more gamelike the task, the better.

Instructional Strategies for the Actual-Spontaneous Learner

The lecture approach will generally be the most ineffective method to use with the ASL. To sit passively and pay attention is not his or her way.

A discussion approach can be effective if it is fast-paced. A hands-on experience will satisfy his or her need for sensation and immediacy. Highly structured assignments that require setting long-range goals or extensive planning are not likely to be completed and thus usually prove ineffective. To assign a paper-and-pencil task is the most ineffective approach to use with this type of learner. Expecting him or her to do an extensive amount of workbook exercises or to read and complete questions on the reading is unrealistic. Assigning homework may be a futile gesture and will provide only an arena of conflict for the student and the teacher.

Hands-on exercises are most effective, and the more gamelike a task the better.

Actual-Routine Learner (38% of Students)

For this temperament type, life is a process of doing what is comfortable and secure combined with a tendency for conforming to and perpetuating what already is. A predisposition exists for observing and preserving the concrete realities of the present. Structure, order, and consistency are important to this student.

The ARL gains knowledge through identifying and memorizing facts and procedures, through repetition and drill, and through sequenced, step-by-step presentation of material. Although this student is uncomfortable in the beginning, as the activities become familiar and the pattern recognizable, he or she will be more comfortable.

If the ARL is asked to invent his or her own procedures or is given vague directions, the student becomes distressed and may begin to falter. When given step-by-step instruction and a routine schedule, the student does quite well. If he or she is required to improvise, guess, or create something on the spot, this student experiences a great deal of difficulty. His or her way is to plan, prepare, and practice; to do otherwise goes against his or her nature. The example for each of the exercises should help this type of student, but the ARL may have difficulty with some of the exercises that ask to figure out various patterns. Doing an exercise as part of the classroom structure supports this student.

Doing the *right* things is as important to ARLs as having the correct answers. Because few correct answers exist in bodywork practice and the textbooks emphasize decision making, this student can become uncomfortable with the activities that are based more on a thought process. To help this type of learner, examples follow.

Instructional Strategies for the Actual-Routine Learner

The ARL needs a great deal of structure and will do best when lessons are presented sequentially in increments that make sense. A lecture approach is effective as long as it is well organized, with the major points being clearly delineated.

Sitting, listening, and taking notes for a long time are done with ease. If this student is presented with an outline to follow, he or she will be most responsive. Additionally, repetition of material is preferred.

Because this student needs to know exactly what the teacher expects, he or she will do best with highly structured exercises. The ARL will be less responsive to role-playing, or dramatization, or any type of exercise that requires him or her to be inventive or spontaneous.

Conceptual-Specific Learner (12% of Students)

Students with this temperament appreciate acquiring knowledge and competence for its own sake or the strategic advantage such knowledge can give an individual or group. A predisposition exists for the abstract with an orientation toward the future.

These learners are naturally curious and generally skeptical.

The CSL places a high value on intellectual achievement. When ideas and analyzing a situation come into play, he or she displays a great deal of patience with the process. Problem solving is highly valued by this type.

The CSL wants to be able to understand, explain, predict, and control realities; and because of this trait, he or she can be characterized as the *little scientist.* This student is not usually interested in isolated facts but wants to use theories and principles in the overall explanation of the facts.

The CSL needs ample opportunity to experiment, to find answers to questions, and to develop explanations for the things that capture his or her interest. Solving a problem is satisfying to this student; conversely, being unable to solve a problem is distressing. In fact, the teacher may need to help these students come to terms with the fact that they will not find the answer to everything.

Learning concrete information or following a routine task will hold little interest for this type of learner.

Instructional Strategies for the Conceptual-Specific Learner

The CSL is comfortable with a logical, didactic presentation of material. Lectures are effective with this student as long as the material is presented in a concise and coherent manner. If the material is repetitious, he or she will become impatient, and attention will wander. Because this student usually has many questions, having a question-and-answer period can be productive, either during or after a presentation.

Being an independent learner, the CSL will enjoy assignments that allow him or her to pursue personal inspirations.

CSLs tend to dislike formal written assignments, preferring to spend their time inquiring into a problem.

Assignments that call for collecting and classifying facts and ideas and that provide the opportunity for inventing, discovering, and designing will be well received. The types of exercises that will be most effective involve some type of problem solving or decision making. He or she will also like brainstorming exercises and seems to enjoy a good debate.

Conceptual-Global Learner (12% of Students)

For students with this temperament, relationships, self-actualization, and developing the potential of people around them are most important.

Born with a predisposition for the abstract, global, and personal, CGLs focus on human potential, ethics, culture, quality of life, metaphysics, and personal growth. These types appreciate metaphor and story telling. Activities need to be meaningful.

The CGL is interested more in conceptualization than in actualization, more in what might be than in what was or is. This learner looks deeply and intensely for the truly meaningful. He or she wants to understand what is important about the facts and what their significance is in the world, not necessarily what they are.

These students are fascinated by people's beliefs and attitudes: what they think, what they want, how they feel, and how they respond.

Instead of using articulated principles and step-by-step solutions, he or she tends to use spontaneous hunches and impressions. When considering facts, the student is looking to confirm impressions rather than attending to the isolated facts themselves.

Instructional Strategies for the Conceptual-Global Learner

An individualized and personalized approach is most effective with the CGL. He or she enjoys interaction and will be enthusiastic as long as a personal focus exists. For instance, when using the lecture method, the presenter can maintain the CGL's involvement by occasionally making eye contact or by providing opportunities for comments or questions.

The style of presentation is also important. Unlike the ASL, the CGL does not want to be entertained, but wants rather to be *moved* by the presentation. If the presenter has a monotone voice and displays a flat affect, the CGL will become bored and inattentive. If the material is presented with enthusiasm, if the presenter is dramatic, and if personal illustrations are used, the CGL will be stimulated and motivated.

Because this type of student enjoys communicating, group discussions will appeal to him or her. Small group discussions will be preferred over large group discussions because they provide more opportunity for personal interaction.

This student will prefer writing a play or recording a story on tape rather than completing a workbook or filling in answers to questions. He or she will also like the opportunity to work independently, as well as cooperatively.

Exercises will be appealing to the CGL as long as they provide him or her the opportunity to interact cooperatively with peers.

APPRECIATING DIVERSITY

Both teachers and students benefit from becoming aware of and learning to appreciate the different personality styles and learning patterns. Such an understanding would not only help him or her have better overall rela-

tionships, but also would help him or her use personal strengths and improve areas of weakness.

Knowing what each type of learner brings to the classroom and how each type typically reacts toward others and what he or she expects from them would be valuable for students. This awareness and appreciation of diversity serve the student and teacher not only in the classroom, but also in the professional world.

- The ASL brings fun and laughter to the classroom.
- The ARL brings to the classroom an interest in social structure, tradition, custom, rules, and routines.
- The CSL brings to the classroom an interest in science and in technical know-how, as well as a natural curiosity and orientation toward the future.
- The CGL brings to the classroom a strong interest in and ability to create a warm, humanistic, enjoyable atmosphere.

The combination of everyone and the diversity of us all provides balance. An analogy can be made to the homeostatic process of the body. A wise instructor will encourage students with different learning styles to work together.

Various tools are available to help determine an individual learning style. This information is based on the MBTI and the Keirsey Bates application of this instrument to temperament and learning style. Obtaining the text used as references would be beneficial in developing this instructor's manual to further expend the understanding of the diversity of the learning experience.

CLINICAL REASONING AND PROBLEM SOLVING

One of the most important traits of a competent professional is the ability to reason though situations to make appropriate decisions, combined with the ability to maintain accurate and thoughtful written records.

Charting involves keeping a written record of professional interactions. Effective charting is more than simply writing down what takes place; it is a clinical reasoning methodology that emphasizes a problem-solving approach to client care. Graduates of programs that teach therapeutic massage are increasingly being employed in the traditional health care system. These individuals bring a firm grounding in complementary modalities. This increase in acceptance by the health care system necessitates developing an outcome-based approach with the ability to gather and analyze data based on goals, develop treatment plans, and operate within a multidisciplinary team plan concept. Being able to justify actions taken on behalf of the client is important. Although these processes may seem different than anatomy, physiology, and pathology, the practical application of material presented in these texts is the component that brings the anatomy, physiology, and pathology information into a concrete usage format for the student. Without this link, anatomy and physiology are often seen as nothing more than a collection of information, and skill application as presented in *Mosby's Fundamentals of Therapeutic Massage* are separate from the sciences. Nothing can be further from the truth.

To help the instructor convey the importance of clinical reasoning and problem solving, this thread is woven through the entire text of both. Each time the student encounters clinical-reasoning activities, they should become more and more familiar so that at the end of the study, the graduate will have developed the habit of processing. This process is fully integrated in Chapter 15 of the textbook as 20 complex case studies are presented.

Charting is the written record of the client process and progress. Charting is also a reflection of the practitioner's ability to gather and analyze data and carry the process through to implementation.

To chart effectively, a practitioner needs a knowledge base of medical terms, abbreviations, and anatomy and physiology in both balanced and imbalanced states of functioning. The instructor must understand the physiologic effects of each massage intervention. Assessment procedures identify deviations from the norm. Information obtained during assessment provides the basis for developing a care plan and identifying contraindications, including more gray areas of cautions and evidence of the need for referral.

SOAP Note Charting

In a problem-oriented medical record (POMR), the acronym SOAP (subjective, objective, analysis [assessment], and plan) defines the four standard parts of the written account of the session. Many other charting systems may be used, but each of these models has similar components to SOAP. Because this process is highly recognized at this time and is easily adapted to other charting models, it has been chosen for the model in this text.

A problem-solving charting model consists of collecting data before beginning to identify the client's problems, (outcome goals). The database consists of all the available information that contributes to the therapeutic interaction. In addition, a history-taking interview with the client and other pertinent people, information from a physical assessment, prior records, health care treatment orders, and any additional relevant sources of information are included.

The initial history interview provides information pertaining to the client's reason for contact, descriptive profile of the person, family illness history, history of current condition and past illnesses, an account of the client's current health practices, and the client's goals for the intervention.

The physical assessment makes up the second part of the database. The extent and depth of the assessment varies from setting to setting, practitioner to practitioner, and according to the situation of the client. Practitioners of therapeutic massage generally use some sort of physical assessment process that looks for bilateral symmetry and variations from it; restricted, exaggerated, painful, or otherwise altered movement patterns; palpation to identify changes in tissue texture, temperature, energy changes, and areas of tenderness; and the use of various manual tests to differentiate soft tissue from joint dysfunction, visceral function, and so on.

The process of gathering this information from the client on the first visit is often called an *intake procedure.* In the textbook is an informed-consent process that essentially provides the client with sufficient information about the qualifications of the professional, general rules and regulations of the professional practice structure, financial and time considerations, referral options for alternative interventions that might be as effective, and much more. Thoroughly investigating the structure and legalities of informed-consent processes would benefit the instructor.

Next, the collected information is analyzed. Each problem that is identified represents a conclusion or decision resulting from examination, investigation, and analysis of the collected data. A problem is defined as anything that causes concern to the client or caregiver, including physical abnormalities, physiologic disturbances, and socioeconomic and spiritual issues. Instead of working to resolve the problems, the client's goals might be the focus. In this regard, wellness and health-enhancing processes such as stress management and relaxation are implemented. A decision is then made about an intervention plan. The action taken and its effectiveness and outcome are recorded in progressive fashion, from session to session, often in what is called a SOAP note.

The SOAP pattern is as follows:

S—Subjective data, information collected from the client and the client's point of view

O—Objective data, acquired from inspection, palpation, tests, and methodology (what was actually done) of the session

A—Analysis or assessment of the subjective and objective data and of the effectiveness of the interventions and actions taken

P—The plan, including the methodology for intervention and progressive sessions

Students often have the most difficulty with the analysis, which is the core of any decision, problem-solving, or clinical-reasoning process. These individuals often avoid a logical outcome and the pro-and-con analysis of the methods being considered. These students also sometimes have difficulty with analysis of effectiveness and benefit of the modality and the procedures used during a session. Another common mistake is for the student to consider opinion or suppositions as facts when in reality they are reflections of internal brainstorming about what all the information might mean. Objectifying some of the subjective experiences that the client reports is also difficult. For example, students often use ambiguous terms such as *tense, tight,* or *client wants to relax,* but what these terms mean remains undefined. Scales of 1 to 10 or other measurements assist in the analysis of *before* and *after* to ascertain benefit during the analysis process. Some students, though strong in the pro-and-con analysis, might have a tendency to avoid considering the impact of the methods on the broader basis of human experience. Because of these inherent problems with decision making, a model for effective record keeping that leads the student through a step-by-step process is beneficial. This type of model is presented and reinforced throughout.

The components of A-analysis processes are:

1. What are the facts?
   - What is considered normal or balanced function?
   - What has happened?
   - What caused the imbalance?
   - What was done or is being done?
   - What has worked or not worked?
2. What are the possibilities?
   - What is my intuition suggesting?
   - What are the possible patterns of dysfunction?
   - What are the possible contributing factors?
   - What are possible interventions?
   - What might work?
   - What are other ways to look at the situation?
   - What does the data suggest?
3. What is the logical progression of the symptom pattern, contributing factors, and current behaviors?
   - What are the logical cause and effect of each intervention identified and a possibility?
   - What are the pros and cons of each intervention suggested?
   - What are the consequences of not acting?
   - What are the consequences of acting?
4. For each intervention being considered, what would be the impact on the people involved: client, practitioner, and other professionals working with the client?
   - How does each person involved feel about the possible interventions?
   - Does the practitioner feel qualified to work with such situations?
   - Does a feeling of cooperation and agreement exist between all parties involved?

All the preceding questions are guides to encourage the reasoning process.

Care or Treatment Plan Development

Once the analysis is complete, a decision needs to be made about what the care or treatment plan will be. This information is developed first in the initial treatment plan structure when the following questions are answered:

1. What are the long- and short-term goals of the intervention process?
2. What are the objective measurable outcomes that indicate the goals have been reached?
3. Is the professional qualified to work with the situation, or is referral or supervision required?
4. What is the expected duration and frequency of the intervention to reach the goals? This information is typically given as an estimate of the number of total sessions and how often the sessions would occur—such as 10 sessions on a weekly basis.
5. What is the estimated cost per session and for the total intervention?
6. What types of modalities should be used to achieve the goals?

This initial treatment plan is the professional's best educated guess of what might occur. Although the plan evolves and changes somewhat as the process takes place, in general, the sessions should follow the plan on which the client agreed.

In the P-plan section of SOAP, the details of the initial treatment plan are implemented, reevaluated, and adjusted as necessary in an ongoing session-to-session basis, setting the stage for the next session with the client.

ACHIEVING COMPETENCY

Being able to apply what is learned comes from the reasoning and problem-solving process. With this ability, the information learned from the study of anatomy and physiology combined with practical application becomes alive and practical. Therapeutic massage professionals become able to justify the efficacy and value of the services they provide. Effective work with clients becomes an ongoing learning process of assessment, determination intervention procedures, analysis of effectiveness by a post-assessment process, and progress made from session to session. Even in the most basic session, in which the client's goal is simply pleasure and relaxation, decisions must still be made on how to best encourage the body to respond to meet this goal. Because these texts are developed on a reasoning model, incorporating this thread into the instructional pattern, building a bridge between science and technical application, is easy. Textbooks need both teachers and students to come alive. *Mosby's Essential Sciences* is primarily a science text; however, it is written in competency-based style to support integrating the scientific information with the skill-based information in *Mosby's Fundamentals of Therapeutic Massage.*

The first part of this instructor's manual has presented an overview of the structure of the textbook, suggestions for using the text, competency-based instruction guidelines, general information about learning styles, and detailed information about teaching a clinical reasoning process and other professional skills. The following chapters focus on instructional support for the individual chapters of the core textbook.

WORKS CONSULTED

Giovannoni LC, Barens LV, Cooper SA: *Introduction to temperament,* Huntington Beach, Calif, 1990, Telos Publications.

Golay K: *Learning patterns and temperament styles,* Fullerton, Calif, 1982, Manas Systems.

Guild PB, Garger S: *Marching to different drummers,* Alexandria, Virg, 1996, Association of Supervision and Curriculum Development.

Keirsey D, Bates M: *Please understand me: character and temperament types,* Del Mar, Calif, 1984, Prometheus Nemesis.

Foundations of Therapeutic Applications of Touch

▼ CONTENT OUTLINE

▼ INSTRUCTOR OBJECTIVES

1. Describe professional touch.
2. Distinguish between professional and nonprofessional forms of touch.
3. Discuss factors that influence the communication of touch.
4. Identify factors that constitute appropriate and inappropriate touch in the professional setting.
5. Assist the student in identifying his or her personal responses to touch.
6. Discuss the influence of personal touch responses during professional interactions.
7. Explain the rich heritage and history of therapeutic massage.
8. Trace the general historical progression of massage from ancient times to the present.
9. Explain the influence of historical events on the current development of therapeutic massage.

CHAPTER SUMMARY

Chapter 1 begins the study of therapeutic massage by exploring concepts of professional touch. An understanding of the power of touch as a therapeutic tool and a means of communication is essential for the massage professional. Various factors influence the application of and receptivity to touch, as well as the therapeutic benefits of touch.

The chapter continues with the historical perspectives of touch as the therapeutic modality of massage, highlighting the events that seem to have the greatest relevance to current trends in therapeutic massage.

The assumption has been made that further study of the anatomy and physiology of skin would take place as part of comprehensive anatomy and physiology studies, such as that provided in the textbook *Mosby's Essential Sciences for Therapeutic Massage: Anatomy, Physiology, Biomechanics, and Pathology*, second edition.

CHAPTER HIGHLIGHTS AND POINTS FOR DISCUSSION

Discuss the following questions:
- Education involves both asking questions and determining answers. Because many questions have multiple answers, what is the truth?
- What is the importance of developing the ability to make a thoughtful choice or decision about which solution is best in a particular situation? How does this ability influence the professional application of touch?
- What is the significance of touch?
- What is professional touch?
- What motivates me to study therapeutic massage?
- What is therapeutic?
- How am I served by touching others?

PROFESSIONAL TOUCH

Professional touch is skilled touch delivered to achieve a specific outcome. The recipient reimburses the professional for services rendered. Discuss touch as a profession. Why would a person want to purchase massage? How does payment influence aspects of professional touch?

Healing pertains to restoration of well being. Therapeutic applications promote a healing environment.

We must be touched to survive. Touch is a hunger that needs to be fed, not just for well being, but also for the very essence of our survival.

Scientific technology has now enabled us to describe some of the physiologic responses to touch, such as changes in concentration of hormones, alterations in central and peripheral nervous system activity, and regulation of body rhythms.

Discuss the difference between healing as a primary motivation for professional touch and providing professional services using touch.

Touch as Communication

In many ways, touch is a more emotionally powerful form of communication than verbal communication. The communication of touch is influenced by personal, family, and cultural contexts. Discuss each of the following influences on the interpretation of touch:
- Culture
- Gender
- Age
- Life events
- Spiritual beliefs
- Diversity

Discussing cultural orientations to touch in generalities or implying that all people from a specific culture hold

to similar customs is inappropriate. Similarly, similar difficulties occur when trying to stereotype by gender, age, life events, or spiritual beliefs. On any given day, or even at any given moment, need, desire, interpretation, and appropriateness of touch given and received can change.

Professional Classifications of Touch

Discuss the forms of inappropriate and appropriate touch and the way in which the professional environment influences when touch is appropriate.

Forms of Inappropriate Touch
- Hostile or aggressive touch. This type of touch interaction occurs when a potential for conflict or a power struggle exists.
- Erotic or sexual touch. The *intention* of this type of touch is sexual arousal and expression. Complex physiologic, mental, and spiritual aspects from both the client and the practitioner influence the ideas of erotic touch. *Erotic feelings should never be acted on with clients.*

  Inherent in many forms of massage and bodywork is the pleasure of being touched, which should not be confused with erotic touch.

Body Areas of Touch Sensitivity
The more emotionally or physically "charged" a body area is, the more the person may feel insecure, anxious, fearful, threatened, connected emotionally, intimate, or aroused when touched in this area.

Some body areas are considered taboo or "no touch zones" in terms of professional bodywork touch. Orifices including the anus, genitals, mouth, ears, and nose have the highest level of taboo in most societies. The ventral (flexor) or front of the body, including the breasts, is more "touch charged" than the dorsal surfaces (extensors). The trunk of the body is more "charged" than the limbs. The head is also a sensitive area to touch. Areas of an individual's body that have undergone trauma, such as during an accident or surgery, carry more emotional charge and therefore are more sensitive to interpretation of the appropriateness of touch.

Discuss why the massage professional would need to understand "touch charged" body areas.

Forms of Appropriate Touch
Nontherapeutic forms of touch often encountered include the following:
- Inadvertent touch
- Socially stereotyped touch
- Touch that communicates information
- Therapeutic forms of touch is considered
- Touch technique

Uniqueness of Touch

Subjective and Objective Quality of Touch

Subjective qualities refer to the aspects experienced, and objective quality refers to the aspects that can be measured. A specific touch experience is difficult to replicate because it is extremely multifaceted. The experience of touching and being touched seems to extend beyond words and verbalization and beyond the skin, nervous system, and endocrine system to the soul.

The desire for physical contact is an instinctive and physiologic need for well being. The concrete experience of caring is most often conveyed through touch. This knowing or "felt sense" that both the client and the practitioner experience is often internalized through professional touch and our willingness as practitioners to be personally open enough to share the experience with the client and professional enough to respect the client and maintain the focus of the experience for the client.

Discuss the subjective and objective qualities of touch.

HISTORICAL PERSPECTIVES

Massage History

Understanding professional structured therapeutic touch requires the exploration of historical influences and the evolution of massage from its ancient foundations to future projections.

Knowledge of history helps professionals develop a sense of professional identity and pride in their profession. Historical perspectives help a profession discover its strengths and weaknesses.

Discuss how history supports professional identity.

Although therapeutic massage has strong roots in Chinese folk medicine, it has much in common with other healing traditions as well. The endurance of massage over the centuries is remarkable. Current trends suggest that the use of massage and body-related therapies is increasing for stress reduction and chronic musculoskeletal problems. Research continues to validate the benefits of massage. After years of struggle for acceptance and validation, massage therapy moved into the mainstream in the mid-1990s. The future direction of massage therapy depends on a commitment to professional ideals.

Discuss the events from the following time line and compare historical events with current trends in therapeutic massage.

Time Line Dates

2000 BC	The art of massage is first mentioned in writing.
460-377 BC	Hippocrates of Cos is the first in Greek medicine to specifically describe the medical benefits of anointing and massage.
25 BC-50 AD	Aulus Cornelius Celsius, a native Roman physician, is credited with compiling *De Medicina*.
129-199	A Greek physician, Claudius Galenus, known as Galen, contributes written material on early manual medicine.
589-617	Duration of Sui dynasty during which knowledge of massage and its applications were already well established in medicine.
1478	*De Medicina* is published using the newly invented Gutenberg printing press.
1517-1590	Ambrose Paré uses massage techniques for joint stiffness and wound healing after surgery.
1776-1839	Per Henrik Ling is given credit for developing Swedish massage.
1837	M. LeRon brings the Movement Cure to Russia.
1839-1909	Dr. Johann Mezger of Holland is given credit for bringing massage to the scientific community.
1852-1943	John Harvey Kellogg, founder of the Battle Creek Sanitarium, writes dozens of articles and two textbooks on massage and hydrotherapy.
1856	Two brothers, Charles Fayette Taylor and George Henry Taylor, introduce the Swedish Movement to the United States.
1879	Douglas Graham writes a history of massage.
1880	Mary Putnam Jacobi and Victoria A. White, medical physicians and professors of medicine in New York City, research the benefits of massage and ice packs in the management of anemia.
1886	Charles K. Mills, a prominent neurologist and massage advocate in Philadelphia, criticizes the uneven quality of lay practitioners of massage.
1894	Massage scandals are uncovered by a commission of inquiry of the British Medical Association in the *British Medical Journal*.
1894	The Society of Trained Masseuses is created.
Early 1900s	Randolph Stone, an American physician, creates polarity therapy.

1916	Dr. James B. Mennell divides the effects of massage into two categories: mechanical and reflex actions.
1918	Polio epidemic renews interest in massage.
1920	Chartered Society of Massage and Medical Gymnastics is created.
1920s	Elizabeth Dicke develops connective tissue massage; Emil and Estrid Vodder develop lymph drainage or manual lymphatic drainage.
1932	Mary McMillan, a lay practitioner, publishes *Massage and Therapeutic Exercise.*
1934	Reich settles in the United States and is considered by many to be the founder of psychotherapeutic body techniques.
Early 1940s	Licensing for physical therapy begins.
1943	The American Association of Masseurs and Masseuses is created.
Late 1940s; early 1950s	James Cyriax publishes the first edition of *Textbook of Orthopedic Medicine.*
1950s	Francis Tappan and Gertrude Beard write important articles and books on massage techniques.
1956	Margaret Knott and Dorothy Voss publish *Proprioceptive Neuromuscular Facilitation.*
1960	President John F. Kennedy emphasizes importance of physical fitness, beginning interest in sports massage.
1960s	The Humanist Movement begins.
1970s	Acupressure receives attention.
Late 1980s	Ronald Melzack publishes a theory of hyperstimulation analgesia in *Clinics in Anesthesiology* to explain endorphin release. This theory was the first in recent decades inspired by findings related to massage.
Late 1980s	The organization Associated Bodywork and Massage Professionals is formed.
1990s	David Palmer formalizes the concepts of on-site or chair massage.
1991	The Touch Research Institute is created; The National Institutes of Health establishes the Office of Alternative Medicine.
1992	National Certification Examination for Therapeutic Massage and Bodywork is first administered.
1993	*The New England Journal of Medicine* reports the use of alternative and complementary forms of health care.
1994	*Alternative Medicine: Expanding Medical Horizons: A Report to the National Institutes of Health on Alternative Medical System and Practiced in the United States* is published.

1995-present Research information about therapeutic massage continues to increase, promoting increased interest on the use of therapeutic massage.

Ask the question: What do you see as the future and how well you will prepare yourself to respond to the changes.

MULTIPLE-CHOICE TEST BANK

_____ 1. Touch as a part of healing interventions:
   a. Developed from multiple cultures
   b. Is based solely on Chinese folk medicine
   c. Was first written approximately 2000 years ago
   d. Did not become popular with physicians until the 1400s

_____ 2. Professional forms of appropriate touch include:
   a. Socially stereotyped touch and aggressive touch
   b. Erotic touch and inadvertent touch
   c. Touch technique and hostile touch
   d. Touch technique and touch that communicates information

_____ 3. Which of the following affects the communication of touch most?
   a. Age and professional attire
   b. Culture and life events
   c. Methodology and gender
   d. Spirituality and training

_____ 4. Hippocrates, a Greek physician:
   a. Endorsed the use of massage for all health conditions
   b. Recommended that assistants, not physicians, perform massage
   c. Was taught massage by Galen
   d. Described the medical benefits of massage

_____ 5. Per Henrik Ling:
   a. Used French terms to describe massage methods
   b. Used many medical terms to describe his work
   c. Combined strokes and gymnastic movements in his work
   d. Was readily accepted by the medical community

_____ 6. The massage scandals of 1894:
  a. Exposed an inconsistent system of education
  b. Did not pertain to private physicians who trained therapists
  c. Were not caused by improper school recruitment tactics
  d. Dealt only with illicit massage

_____ 7. Current historians give credit to:
  a. The Germans for promoting and teaching massage to the blind
  b. Albert Hoffa's writings on classical massage techniques
  c. Sister Kenny for connective tissue work
  d. Elizabeth Dicke and Maria Ebner for using massage in treating polio

_____ 8. The development of manual lymphatic drainage is credited to:
  a. Louise K. Despard
  b. Emil Vodder
  c. Mary McMillan
  d. Max Bohm

_____ 9. One of the most influential massage researchers of current times is:
  a. Ronald Melzack
  b. Dorothy Voss
  c. David Palmer
  d. Dr. Tiffany Field

_____ 10. Future trends suggest that the massage profession is changing in which of the following ways?
  a. Professional massage is becoming more sophisticated, requiring increased education.
  b. The rate of acceptance for massage is slow but steady.
  c. Massage professionals will work primarily outside the health care environment.
  d. Multiple employment opportunities within the service/wellness area of massage will decrease, and jobs in managed health care will increase.

_____ 11. The practice of acupuncture involves:
  a. The stimulation of specific points along the body, usually by the insertion of tiny, solid needles
  b. The stimulation of specific points along the body, usually by the pressing of the thumb into the point
  c. The stimulation of broad points along the body, usually by accomplishing a series of ever deepening compressive strokes
  d. Using counter initiation, such as scraping, cutting, or burning of skin to relieve pain

_____ 12. Professionalism is defined as:
  a. An occupation that helps people
  b. A service provided for others
  c. An intricate system that is structured and very systematic
  d. Adherence to professional status, methods, standards, and character.

_____ 13. One of the prominent reasons that Ling's work had a difficult time being accepted was because:
  a. He worked only with healthy people.
  b. He used poetic and mystic language in his writings.
  c. He based his work on newly discovered knowledge of the circulation of the blood and lymph.
  d. The primary focus was on gymnastics.

_____ 14. What is the massage trend that developed in 1991 that supported acceptance for the benefits of massage?
  a. Increase in valid research
  b. Deregulation of massage education
  c. Decrease in influential women in the profession
  d. Resistance to integrating massage into traditional health care settings.

CHAPTER 2

Professionalism and Legal Issues

▼INSTRUCTOROBJECTIVES

1. Define and model (the way in which you, as an instructor, present yourself) professionalism in the classroom.
2. Compare therapeutic massage and professional development criteria.
3. Describe the two professional development trends for therapeutic massage.
4. Define *therapeutic massage.*
5. Explain the differences and similarities of various approaches to massage and bodywork.
6. Clarify the seven basic approaches to therapeutic massage and bodywork.
7. Classify a massage method according to its fundamental physiologic response.
8. Define a scope of practice for therapeutic massage.
9. Explain the scope of practice of various health and service professionals.
10. Explain what constitutes the practice of medicine.
11. Explain the difference between medical rehabilitative massage and wellness massage.
12. Guide students in developing a scope of practice for massage that respects that of other professionals.
13. Explain the code of ethics and standards of practice concerns for therapeutic massage.
14. Explain and demonstrate how to complete an informed consent process.
15. Explain the nine components of informed consent.
16. Explore criteria that determine whether a client can provide informed consent for a massage.
17. Explain the importance of written client information materials to support the informed consent process.
18. Demonstrate the process of completing two different types of informed consent forms.
19. Discuss the process of establishing and maintaining client confidentiality.
20. Demonstrate the process of completing a release of information form.
21. Discuss and explore professional boundaries and the therapeutic relationship.
22. Guide the student in developing strategies for maintaining professional boundaries with clients.
23. Guide the student in exploring personal prejudices, fears, and limitations that may interfere with the ability to provide the best care for a client.
24. Develop criteria that allow the student to help a client recognize personal boundaries in the massage process.
25. Define and recognize potential transference and countertransference issues.
26. Explain the professional power differential.
27. List criteria that create dual or multiple roles.
28. Discuss with students the potential for a client to have feelings of intimacy with the massage professional.
29. Discuss and model methods to diffuse sexual feelings during the massage session.
30. Present criteria that the student can use to recognize and avoid sexual misconduct activities.
31. Present and demonstrate a problem-solving approach to enhance ethical decision making.
32. Implement an eight-part decision-making process.
33. Present basic communications skills that allow the student to listen effectively and deliver an I-message.
34. Present criteria that allow the student to identify a person's preferred communication pattern.
35. Teach and use an I-message to both deliver information and listen reflectively.
36. Explain and model the process of following a suggested communication pattern for resolving ethical dilemmas and conflict.
37. Identify three barriers to effective communication.
38. Identify legal and credentialing concerns of the massage professional.
39. Explain the difference between government and private credentials.
40. Present criteria that allow the student to determine whether a credentialing program is valid.
41. Explain the basic role of local and state legislation and its influence on therapeutic massage.
42. Provide guidance so that the student is able to contact local or state or provincial governments to obtain information about legislation pertinent to the practice of therapeutic massage.
43. Discuss criteria that will allow the student to identify and report unethical conduct of colleagues.
44. Explain the four steps involved in reporting unethical behavior.

CHAPTER SUMMARY

This chapter defines *therapeutic massage,* identifies the types of professional services a massage practitioner can legally and ethically provide, and establishes guidelines for conduct in the professional setting. This information base provides the structure to make appropriate professional and ethical decisions, which is essential to develop the level of professionalism required for a successful therapeutic massage practice. My years of professional experience confirm that when a massage professional encounters difficulty in the professional setting, it is seldom a problem with a technical skill and almost always an ethical dilemma. Acquiring the decision-making skills used with the problem-solving model and developing effective communication skills are likely some of the most valuable tools contained in this text.

CHAPTER HIGHLIGHTS AND POINTS FOR DISCUSSION

The subjects of ethics and professionalism are of great importance to the bodywork profession. The ambiguity of ethics blends with the concreteness of professionalism and the standards of practice to provide a basis for ethical decision making in any profession.

Discuss the following general criteria of professionals. In general, a professional is one who has:

1. A specialized body of knowledge
2. A long period of training
3. An orientation toward service
4. A commonly accepted code of ethics
5. Legal recognition through certification or licensure
6. A professional association

Discuss the ways in which the therapeutic massage professional meets these criteria.

The therapeutic massage profession has not yet agreed on a professional career name. Establishing a unique professional identity is difficult when we do not know our name.

Discuss whether massage professionals are technicians, practitioners, or therapists and what each term implies.

In the last few years, as the popularity of therapeutic massage has increased, the profession has seen an expansion of styles and systems (Box 2-1 in the text). The term *bodywork* has been used to describe the scope of these developments. As the individual systems have emerged, a difference in the styles has developed. The overlap of these methods, however, reveals a fundamental uniformity in all of the work.

Discuss the overlapping aspects of bodywork systems.

Discuss why the profession must begin to standardize terminology to avoid confusion about the various styles and systems of massage.

The definition of massage needs to include all the methods that the various systems use (Box 2-2 in the text). In addition, the definition of *therapeutic massage* depends on individual laws and the definition of *massage* included in these laws.

Discuss the importance and limitations of the definition of *massage*.

A scope of practice defines the knowledge base and practice parameters of a profession. Each individual within a particular profession acquires a specific knowledge base and needs to define a personal scope of practice.

A scope of practice that has been legally adopted through legislation defines, as well as limits, the ability to practice massage. Respectful practice of therapeutic massage limits the scope of practice so as not to encroach on other professional scopes of practice.

Each professional also has personal limits to the scope of practice. These limits involve the type and extent of education received, personal biases, life experiences, specific interests in terms of the type of client served, and any physical limitations such as size and endurance levels. Professional limits are valid and valuable; they allow us to set and maintain boundaries that support each professional in the most successful practice structure.

Discuss how the student would first define the scope of practice and then how individual scopes of practice evolve with increased education, experience, and so forth.

When a client expresses distress, shares personal information, or requests specific information, first identify whether the issue is most specifically a body, mind, or spirit issue. If a mental or spiritual issue is raised, use listening skills and acknowledge the situation, but do not attempt to problem solve or provide professional intervention. If the situation is physical, determine whether the nature of the information falls within the scope of therapeutic bodywork and then respond accordingly.

Discuss the criteria that a student can use to make this determination.

The severity or complex nature of the situation will indicate whether simple listening, without the addition of advice, is sufficient or whether a professional referral is indicated. Discuss the development of referral networks.

Understanding the functioning realms of people and the scope of practice of massage and bodywork helps the professional establish an ethical practice and begin the discovery of the therapeutic process.

Ethics defines the behavior we expect of ourselves and others and what society expects of a profession. Ethics has social, professional, and personal dimensions; ethical behavior must be a dynamic process of reflection and revision.

Discuss similarities and differences of cultural, professional, and personal ethics.

The purpose of practicing our profession ethically is to promote and maintain the welfare of the client. A professional code of ethics is a set of moral norms adopted by a professional group to direct value-laden choices in a manner consistent with professional responsibility.

Discuss how the following principles guide professional ethical behavior:

- Respect: esteem and regard for clients, other professionals, and self
- Client's autonomy or self-determination: the freedom to decide and the right to sufficient information to make a decision
- Veracity: the right to the objective truth
- Proportionality: benefit must outweigh the burden of treatment
- Nonmaleficence: doing no harm and preventing harm from happening
- Beneficence: contributing to well being
- Confidentiality: respect for privacy of information
- Justice: equality

Standards of practice provide specific guidelines and rules to form a concrete professional structure. Because the massage therapy and bodywork profession is still not united in terms of professional affiliation and techniques, providing a code of ethics or agreed-on standards of practice is difficult for the massage professional.

Discuss what might be done about this dilemma.

Informed consent is a protection process for the consumer. Informed consent requires that clients have knowledge of what will occur, that their participation is voluntary, and that they are competent to give consent. Informed consent is an educational procedure that allows clients to make knowledgeable decisions about whether they want to receive a massage, whether they want a particular therapist to work with them, and whether the professional structure, including client rules and regulations, is acceptable to them. Clients must be able to provide informed consent and demonstrate that they understand the information presented to them.

Parents or guardians must provide informed consent for minors. Guardians must provide informed consent for those who are too disabled or otherwise unable to do so.

True informed consent provides the opportunity to evaluate the options and risks involved with each method and requires the massage professional to include information about inherent and potential hazards of the proposed treatment, alternatives, and the likely results if treatment does not occur.

A comprehensive intake procedure, including an informed consent process, is necessary for the client when defined outcomes span a series of sessions.

A *needs assessment,* based on a client history and a physical assessment, is used to form an *initial treatment plan.* The initial treatment plan states therapeutic goals, duration of the sessions, number of appointments necessary to meet the agreed-on goals, costs, general classification of intervention to be used, and the objective progress measurement to identify when goals have been reached. (Procedures for completing forms associated with these procedures are presented in Chapter 3.)

Single or random massage sessions usually do not include a full needs assessment or require treatment plan development. Instead, possible contraindications to massage are identified. The informed consent process informs the client of the limitations a single massage session and the approaches to be used in the single session massage or bodywork experience.

Discuss and model various approaches to providing and obtaining informed consent.

Confidentiality means that a client's information is private and belongs to the client. Confidentiality is built on respect and trust. Client information is never discussed with anyone other than the client without the client's written permission. Client files need to represent the information accurately only as it relates to the service offered.

Discuss the method used to decide what information belongs in client files and what information does not.

During informed consent procedures, clients must understand limits to confidentiality. Information exchanged between professionals requires that the client sign a release of information form. A sample of this form is provided in the text.

The massage professional should have a clear understanding of personal motivation in the therapy setting and carefully maintain professional boundaries. An important first step therefore is to begin the exploration of professional boundaries by looking honestly at our own fears, frustrations, prejudices, biases, and value systems.

Discuss this issue in depth. A thorough discussion is important for all service professionals. The instructor needs to be aware of the complexities of individual student beliefs and provide a balance in both challenging and respecting individual beliefs of the student. The goal is awareness of the influence of such beliefs in the professional setting. The goal is not for the student to probe deeply into the personal process to elicit internal change. Although this result may occur as a part of the process of education, it is not the primary goal of either the instructor or the student.

Clients have the right to refuse the massage practitioner's services. This action is called the *right of refusal.* A client has the right to refuse or stop treatment at any time. When this request is made during treatment, the therapist must comply despite prior consent. Professionals also have right of refusal. Massage professionals may refuse to administer to, massage, or otherwise treat any person if *just and reasonable cause* exists.

Discuss criteria that create just and reasonable cause.

Blurred boundaries create the environment for the development of ethical dilemmas. *Transference* involves the personalization of the professional relationship by the client. *Countertransference* occurs when the professional is unable to separate the therapeutic relationship from personal feelings and expectations for the client and personalizes the therapeutic relationship. Countertransference is often fed by the following personal needs of the therapist:

- The need to fix people
- The need to remove pain and discomfort
- The need to be perfect
- The need to have the answer
- The need to be loved

Discuss the difference between *wanting to* and *needing to* relative to fixing people, removing pain and discomfort, being perfect, having the answer, and being loved.

Peer support and supervision become important for the massage professional dealing with transference and countertransference issues. The professional has the ultimate responsibility for the therapeutic relationship and the direction of the therapeutic process.

A dual or multiple role develops when the professional assumes more than one role in the relationship with the client. Dual and multiple roles are difficult to manage

in the professional relationship and can be a breeding ground for the development of ethical dilemmas.
Discuss various situations that foster dual roles.

Discuss the balance of professional intimacy within the parameters of the therapeutic relationship based on the following criteria.

The massage professional must possess an awareness of the physiologic aspects of therapeutic massage and show how the same techniques of massage that alleviate stress and promote relaxation also stimulate the entire sensory mechanism, which may include a sexual arousal response. Within the parameters of professional ethics, *interacting on a sexual level, whether verbal or physical, is always considered unethical for the client or the practitioner.* However, both client and practitioner must understand why the urges and sensations of sexuality may develop.

Massage practitioners must always be honest with themselves about the development of personal feelings for a client. Remember that a relationship exists and that professional relationships can last a long time. These people become important to us. The touch of a massage professional is *safe* touch.

Discuss how to maintain the therapeutic relationship as a unidirectional focus using the knowledge and skills of the professional to assist the client in achieving therapeutic outcomes.

When ethical dilemmas are difficult to resolve, massage therapists are expected to engage in a conscientious decision-making process that is explicit enough to bear public scrutiny. Decision making includes consideration of the facts, possibilities, logical consequences of cause and effect, and the effect on people. Each decision is unique. A problem-solving model not only leads us through the steps we would more naturally take, but also reminds us to look at important information we might tend to overlook when making a decision.

Discuss and reinforce the importance of decision making.

Supervision involves periodic review of a professional's actions by one who is more experienced in professional practice. The more experienced professional is able to guide, coach, and mentor the one being supervised and help with identifying potential ethical concerns, as well as assist in ethical decision making. Peer support provides a format for discussing, brainstorming, and reflecting on the professional practice. Two or three heads are better than one when working with ethical decision making.

Discuss the importance of supervision and peer support. Discuss how a person supervises himself or herself.

Communication is the act of exchanging thoughts, feelings, and behavior. The strongest message is delivered through the kinesthetic mode, or body language. The tone of the voice is more important than the words that are spoken. The words are the least effective part of the communication pattern. Words have mixed meanings, depending on the definition of the word for each person.

Each person has a preferred method of delivering and receiving information in a style that is most comfortable for him or her. This style is determined by genetic predisposition and conditioning (learning). The processing styles are visual, auditory, and kinesthetic.

Effective listening involves development of focusing skills. A person who is planning what to say next or how to respond cannot listen effectively. Reflective listening includes restating the information to indicate that the message has been received and understood. Active listening may clarify a feeling attached to the message but does not add to or change the message. *Listening does not involve the addition of advice, resolution of the problem presented, or in any other way interjecting information about what was said.* Effective listening occurs when we listen to understand rather than to respond. *Understanding* the message and *agreeing* with the content of the message are not the same thing. I-message patterns require that the four components of information for effective decision making are presented. Refer to Box 2-15 in the text.

When delivering I-messages, it is important to remain pleasant, respectful, and honest and to be aware of one's body language, tone of voice, and quality of touch. After an I-message is delivered, it is important to request a response by using *open-ended questions.* Open-ended questions encourage the sharing of information and cannot be answered easily in one word. These questions begin with the words *where, when, what, how,* and *which.* Avoid why questions because they encourage defensive reactions.

The I-message format can also be an effective listening tool. While listening, organize the information into the following components:

- What happened? (the facts)
- What feelings are being expressed?
- What was the logical outcome?
- What are the possibilities?

When reflectively listening, repeat the information back as follows: "What I heard you say was…." "When… happened, you felt…." "The result was and what you prefer is…." "Did I understand correctly?"

Discuss the many uses of the I-message and open-ended question patterns.

The following series of steps is a suggested pattern for resolving ethical dilemmas:

- Carefully examine the fact, possibilities, logical cause and effects, and personal feelings regarding the situation. Speak with a peer about the situation in a peer review or support context.
- Plan a time to discuss the situation with the person.
- Begin the conversation by identifying the problem as you see it.
- Use the standard I-message format to dispense the information and provide professional disclosure about the inability to work with or be comfortable with the situation.

Discuss how time, old patterns, and avoidance interfere with effective communication. Relate how these issues interfere with conflict management. Relate how these issues interfere with conflict management.

Discuss the importance of the I-message both for delivering information and for effective listening and questioning. Integrate the aspects of conflict management.

Credentials are designations earned by completing an educational or examination process that verifies a certain level of expertise in a given skill. The only credentials required for the practice of therapeutic massage are enacted by the government (Box 2-16 in the text). All other credentials are voluntary. Many massage and bodywork organizations' training programs have developed their own types of credentials. These credentials are valid only in that they indicate a level of professional achievement. A school diploma, which is received after completing the course work, is an example of this type of credential. This process is important for a massage professional, but it is not a legally required credential unless stipulated by law.

Medical massage is supposed to be supervised by licensed medical professionals, and the responsibility for the client's safety rests with the supervising personnel.

Regulations, standards of practice, codes of conduct, scopes of practice, and so forth are methods of setting the rules for cooperative professional relationships.

Discuss the various types of credentials and the advantages and disadvantages of each.

What is the appropriate way to address unethical behavior and violations of standards of practice with colleagues?

Discuss each of the following in relation to unethical behavior by peers:
- Self-reflection
- Peer support and supervision
- Communication with those involved
- Formal reporting

MULTIPLE-CHOICE TEST BANK

_____ 1. Ethics:
   a. Deal only with personal relationships
   b. Should be defined by professional organizations, not individuals
   c. Are concerned with right and wrong judgment
   d. Are the same for each person

_____ 2. A definition of massage:
   a. Is inclusive of all massage methods
   b. Has been agreed on by the profession
   c. Is not affected by massage laws
   d. Is easy to create

_____ 3. The scope of practice for massage:
   a. Allows for the diagnosis and treatment of minor diseases
   b. Allows for the dispensing of medicinal and nutritional advice to healthy people
   c. Allows one level of practice for all massage school graduates
   d. Allows various levels of practice based on educational and training requirements

_____ 4. A code of ethics:
   a. Determines policy for resolving ethical dilemmas
   b. Helps professionals make ethical decisions
   c. Identifies personal values
   d. Provides standards of practice measurement criteria

_____ 5. Informed consent:
   a. Is the responsibility of the client to ask questions regarding quality of care
   b. Is necessary in licensed states to protect the public's health, welfare, and safety
   c. Provides the client with skills to perform appropriate self-help techniques
   d. Provides the client with sufficient information to be able to understand the massage process

_____ 6. A professional boundary:
   a. Defines personal, physical, and emotional space within the therapeutic relationship
   b. Defines only the space of the client in the therapeutic relationship
   c. Defines personal, physical, and emotional space
   d. Defines the limits of scope of practice in legislation

_____ 7. Countertransference concerns:
   a. Personalizing the therapeutic relationship by the client
   b. Obtaining informed consent
   c. Personalizing the therapeutic relationship by the therapist
   d. Objectifying the client's therapeutic goals

_____ 8. An ethical decision-making process includes consideration of:
   a. Facts, possibilities, logical consequences, and impact on people
   b. Facts, possibilities, informed consent, and impact on people
   c. Brainstorming, supervision, investigating pros and cons, and treatment outcomes
   d. Facts, possibilities, logical consequences, and impact on the client

_____ 9. An I-message includes the following components:
   a. Description of the problem and implementation plans
   b. Facts, impact on people, logical cause and effect, and possibilities
   c. Effective listening, open-ended questioning, brainstorming possibilities, and analysis of facts
   d. Visual, auditory, and kinesthetic presentation

_____ 10. Credentials:
   a. Are developed only by legislative bodies
   b. Protect the public's health, welfare, and safety
   c. Are legal documents
   d. Are verification of a certain level of expertise in a given skill

_____ 11. Which of the following is a violation of confidentiality?
   a. Maintaining client records in a secure location
   b. Asking the client questions about work environment
   c. Approaching and speaking to a client in a restaurant
   d. Speaking to a client's chiropractor with appropriate releases

_____ 12. Local legislation controlling the location of a business is:
   a. Licensing
   b. Building codes
   c. DBA
   d. Zoning

_____ 13. A massage professional has been working with a particular client for 12 months. Recently, the client has been experiencing increased difficulties with her family communications. The biggest problem is stress and tension between her son and his father. Discussions during massage are focused on solving this problem. Which of the following best describes this situation?
   a. The massage professional is having difficulty maintaining informed consent.
   b. Scope of practice violations particularity with psychology are occurring.
   c. The client should be referred to either acupuncture of chiropractic.
   d. The client is engaged in countertransference.

_____ 14. Which of the following would be an appropriate disclosure to a client?
   a. The massage professional tells the client that the professional has a cold.
   b. The massage professional tells the client about business or financial concerns.
   c. The massage professional tells the client about mutual acquaintances.
   d. Marital difficulties are revealed to the client.

_____ 15. A massage professional is careful to provide an informed consent process for each client and updates informed consent on a regular basis. Which of the following ethical principles is informed consent following?
   a. Confidentiality
   b. Justice
   c. Proportionality
   d. Client autonomy and self-determination

Medical Terminology for Professional Record Keeping

▼INSTRUCTOROBJECTIVES

1. Identify the three word elements used in medical terms.
2. Combine word elements into medical terms. Use the text in *Mosby's Essential Sciences for Therapeutic Massage: Anatomy, Physiology, Biomechanics, and Pathology,* second edition, Chapter 3, as an additional source.
3. Translate medical terms.
4. Define words by breaking them down into their word elements.
5. Identify common abbreviations.
6. Identify pertinent abbreviations used in health care and their meanings.

7. Demonstrate how to use Appendix A in the textbook to identify indications and contraindications to massage. Pathology sections with Indications/Contraindications are presented throughout *Mosby's Essential Sciences* text.

8. Review relevant anatomy and physiology terminology.

9. Demonstrate the use of medical terminology for effective professional recording keeping. See *Mosby's Essential Sciences* Chapter 3 for charting forms.

10. Present the process of a client intake using sample forms.

11. Implement the clinical reasoning/decision-making model for charting purposes.

12. Explain how to use a problem/goal-oriented charting process.

13. Explain how to chart using a SOAP note format.

CHAPTER SUMMARY

This chapter describes the medical terminology that the massage professional most often encounters, particularly as it relates to charting and record-keeping procedures. To study this chapter, you will need to use a medical dictionary. Exploring medical terminology automatically provides an overview of anatomy and physiology. The chapter is not meant to replace an anatomy and physiology text, but rather to provide a quick reference as record-keeping and charting skills are developed. When used with a standard anatomy and physiology textbook and class instruction, this chapter can help focus the information so that it is more specific to the field of massage. The recommended anatomy and physiology text is *Mosby's Essential Sciences* because it has been developed specifically for massage and bodywork students. However, the information in this chapter is relevant for use with any comprehensive anatomy and physiology book.

CHAPTER HIGHLIGHTS AND POINTS FOR DISCUSSION

Having agreement with regard to terminology is important. Without a common language, we cannot communicate. To be able to communicate with their clients in a common language that both can understand is the responsibility of massage professionals.

Discuss why multiple terms for the same method might have developed.

Discuss difficulties that may occur as a result of differences in terminology.

Medical terms are made up of combined word elements. A term can be interpreted easily by separating the word into its elements. These word elements include prefixes, roots, and suffixes.

Abbreviations are shortened forms of words or phrases. When you use abbreviations in any record keeping, including charting, provide an abbreviation key either on the forms or in a conspicuous place in the file. Using an overabundance of abbreviations makes reading difficult and requires interpretation. Jargon should also be avoided in record keeping.

Demonstrate how to determine the meaning of medical language.

Discuss the use of abbreviations and jargon.

Following is a brief list of common terms and a quick overview of anatomy and physiology. Presenting this information is a good opportunity to justify the importance of anatomy and physiology studies in relation to theory and technique studies.

An *indication* exists when an approach would be beneficial for health enhancement, for treatment of a particular condition, or to support a treatment modality other than massage.

A *contraindication* exists when an approach might be harmful. When contraindications exist, one of the following should occur:

- General avoidance of application—do not massage.
- Regional avoidance of application—massage is permissible, but avoid a particular area.
- Application is performed with caution, usually requiring supervision from appropriate medical or supervising personnel. Massage is permissible, but carefully select the type of methods to be used, duration of the massage, and frequency.

Directional terms are used to describe how one body part relates to another.

The body consists of tissues. A tissue is a collection of specialized cells that perform a special function. *Histo* is a root, meaning tissue. Histology is the study of tissue. The primary tissues of the body are epithelial, connective, muscular, and nervous.

An organ is a collection of specialized tissues. An organ has a specific function or functions but does not act independently of other organs. Organs make up systems.

The body cavities contain the organs and are divided into ventral and dorsal regions. The back or posterior surface of the trunk is also divided into the following regions:

- Cervical region: the neck (seven cervical vertebrae)
- Thoracic region: the chest (twelve thoracic vertebrae)
- Lumbar region: the loin (five lumbar vertebrae)
- Sacral region: the sacrum (five sacral vertebrae that are fused into one bone)
- Coccyx: the tailbone (four coccygeal vertebrae that are fused into one bone)

The skeletal system consists of three elements: bones, cartilage, and ligaments. Chapter 7 in *Mosby's Essential Sciences* focuses on the skeletal system.

Tissues that are contractile make up the muscular system. The three types of muscle tissue include cardiac muscle, smooth muscle, and skeletal muscle. The Muscles chapter, Chapter 9 in *Mosby's Essential Sciences,* is an in depth source for this topic.

Study of the nervous system is important for the massage professional and focuses on the following:
- Central nervous system (CNS)
- Peripheral nervous system (PNS)
- Autonomic nervous system (ANS)

For additional sources, see Chapters 4 and 5 in *Mosby's Essential Sciences.*

The cardiovascular system consists of two parts: the heart and the blood vessels.

The lymphatic system is responsible for several functions and operates in the following ways:
- Returns vital substances, such as plasma protein, to the bloodstream from the tissues of the body
- Assists in maintaining fluid balance by draining fluid from the body tissues
- Helps the body defend against disease-producing substances
- Helps absorb fats from the digestive system

The human body is able to resist organisms or toxins that tend to damage the tissues and organs that make up the body. This ability is called immunity. Nonspecific and specific immunity and the immune system is explained in more depth in *Mosby's Essential Sciences.*

The respiratory system supplies oxygen and removes carbon dioxide from the cells of the body. The two phases of respiration are external and internal.

See the respiratory and the digestive chapter, Chapter 12, in *Mosby's Essential Sciences* for an in-depth explanation of the respiratory system.

The anatomy of the digestive system can be compared with that of a long muscular tube that travels a path through the body (Figure 3-12 in text). The organs of the digestive system break down food and transport food and waste through these muscular tubes.

The endocrine system is composed of glands that produce hormones that are secreted directly into the bloodstream to stimulate cells in a specific way or to set a body function into action. Chapter 6 in *Mosby's Essential Sciences* is devoted to the endocrine system.

The integumentary system consists of the skin and its appendages, including hair and nails. In Chapter 11 of *Mosby's Essential Sciences*, the integumentary system is explained.

Written Records

Appreciating the need to maintain a written record of the professional relationship with a client and focusing on clinical decision making and the records necessary for maintaining a written account of the professional interaction are important.

Record keeping for clients involves the written record of intake procedures, including informed consent, needs assessments (including history and physical assessment), obtaining release of information, and the ongoing process of recording each session, which is called *charting.*

Discuss the importance of maintaining written records. In *Mosby's Essential Sciences*, Chapter 3, Medical Terminology, Charting, and Record Keeping is discussed along with decision making. Additionally, a section on regional terms may be found that are used to designate specific areas of the body.

Therapeutic massage practitioners must be able to gather information effectively, analyze the information to make decisions about the type and appropriateness of a therapeutic intervention, and evaluate and justify the benefits derived from the intervention. Effective charting is more than writing down what happened; it is a clinical reasoning methodology that emphasizes a problem-solving approach to client care.

Review the decision-making process presented in Chapter 2.

Sessions with massage professionals are goal oriented. *Goals* describe desired outcomes.

Goals must be able to be *quantified.* This description means that goals are measured in terms of objective criteria such as time, frequency, 1-to-10 scales, measurable increase or decrease in the ability to perform an activity, or measurable increase or decrease in a sensation, such as relaxation or pain.

Goals also need to be *qualified.* How will we know when the goal is achieved? What will clients be able to do after the goal is reached that they are not able to do now? Before beginning work with a client, the massage professional should gather information on which to build the professional interaction, establish client goals, and develop a plan for achieving the client goals. The result is called a *database.*

Discuss and demonstrate goal setting.

The I-message pattern can be altered slightly to develop effective open-ended questions that support data collection.

The four basic questions are:
- Will you please explain the situation or tell me what happened?
- How did or do you feel about the situation?
- What was the result of the situation in terms of cost, limitations, or changes in activity or performance?
- How would you prefer the situation to be handled, or what would you like to occur?

Provide practice opportunities for the student to use the preceding questions in role-play situations in the classroom.

The history interview provides information pertaining to the client's health history, the reason for contact, a descriptive profile of the person, a history of the current condition, a history of illness and health, and a history of any family illnesses. An account of the client's current health practices is also assessed. The history interview provides the first part of the database.

The physical assessment makes up the second part of the database. Assessment procedures identify both deviations from the norm and effective functioning. After the information is collected, it is analyzed by using these steps:

1. Review the facts and information collected from the database and resource information. Questions that help with this process are:
   - What are the facts?
   - What is considered normal or balanced function?
   - What has happened? (Spell out events.)
   - What caused the imbalance? (Can it be identified?)
   - What was done or is being done?
   - What has worked or not worked?
2. Brainstorm the possibilities. Questions that help with this process are:
   - What are the possibilities? (What might it all mean?)
   - What does my intuition suggest?
   - What are the possible patterns of dysfunction?
   - What are the possible contributing factors?
   - What are possible interventions?
   - What might work?
   - What are other ways to look at the situation?
   - What do the data suggest?
3. Determine the logical outcome of each possibility. Questions that help with this process are:
   - What is the logical progression of the symptom pattern, contributing factors, and current behaviors?
   - What is the logical cause and effect of each intervention identified?
   - What are the pros and cons of each intervention suggested?
   - What are the consequences of not acting?
   - What are the consequences of acting?
4. Determine ways in which people would be affected by each possibility. Questions that help with this process are:
   - In terms of each intervention being considered, what would be the impact on the people involved— client, practitioner, and other professionals working with the client?
   - What does each person involved think about the possible interventions?
   - Is the practitioner within his or her scope of practice to work with such situations?
   - Is the practitioner qualified to work with such situations?
   - Does the practitioner believe that he or she is qualified to work with such situations?
   - Does a sense of cooperation and agreement exist among all parties involved?

Problem areas of focus are then identified, based on a conclusion or decision resulting from examination, investigation, and analysis of the data collected. A problem is defined as anything that causes concern to the client or caregiver, including physical abnormalities, physiologic disturbances, and socioeconomic or spiritually based problems. Realistic and attainable functional outcome goals are established. A *decision* is then made about an intervention or care or treatment plan.

Not all therapeutic goals are in relation to problems. Clients often use massage for health maintenance, stress management, and fulfillment of pleasure needs. The same analysis process is used to determine the methods and approach to best meet client goals.

Provide opportunities for the student to practice the analysis process using role-play with case studies in the text.

After the analysis is complete and problems and goals have been identified, a *decision* must be made about what will be involved in the care or treatment plan. The plan is not an exact protocol that is set in stone, but rather a fluid guideline (the best professional educated guess). As the plan is implemented, it is recorded sequentially session by session in some form of charting process such as SOAP (subjective, objective, assessment/analysis, and plan) notes. The plan is reevaluated and adjusted as necessary.

Discuss, demonstrate, and reinforce the intake process with the students.

Charting is the ongoing record of each client session. A commonly used method of charting is the problem-oriented medical record (POMR). One type of POMR is SOAP charting.

The *key skill* is the ability to rationally and comprehensively reason through a therapeutic interaction.

A charting process can provide the structure necessary to think through a process effectively and develop a written record of the process.

Discuss various charting methods.

When using SOAP note charting, the following pattern is used:

1. **S:** Subjective data are recorded from the client's point of view. Subjective information usually includes:
   - Key symptoms that are quantified and qualified
   - Activities that are affected by the situation, often stated as what can no longer be done or what increase in performance is desired
   - Methods or activities currently being used
2. **O:** Objective data are acquired from inspection, palpation, and testing of any applications. A list of assessment procedures and interventions used during the session is recorded. Objective information usually includes:
   - Physical assessment findings that are significant

- Intervention modalities and locations that were used (Limit specifics to interventions used to work toward treatment goals.)
- General approach used (e.g., connective tissue massage, Swedish massage, neuromuscular massage)
- If not recorded elsewhere, the duration of the session (e.g., 1 hour)

3. **A:** Analysis or assessment of the subjective and objective data is made, as well as analysis of the effectiveness of the intervention and action taken. The most pertinent data are summarized and recorded.

NOTE: **Traditionally in SOAP charting, the *A* stands for assessment. Students are sometimes confused about the difference between physical assessment information that is recorded in the Objective data and the *A*-assessment in the soap model. The latter is actually an *analysis* of the data and effectiveness of the interventions. Therefore this text uses the concept of analysis for the A section of SOAP charting.**

Analysis/Assessment information usually includes the following:

- Subjective and objective changes. Subjective changes relate to clients' experience (e.g., pain is reduced or they feel relaxed). Objective changes are changes that can be measured (e.g., flexion of elbow is increased by 15 degrees). If no change occurs or the condition worsens, this information is also recorded.
- Analysis of which methods were effective and which were not effective (for example, trigger point most effective in increase of flexion of elbow; client indicated that he or she responded best to rhythmic rocking for relaxation; tense and relax methods not effective in reducing pain in shoulder). If the choice as to which methods were effective is unclear, this information should also be recorded (e.g., range of motion in neck increased 25%, but it is unclear which methods were responsible for this change). The analysis/assessment section of the SOAP charting process is the most important area for determining future intervention procedures and communicating process information to other caregivers and insurance companies.

4. **P:** Plan includes developing and recording the methodology for intervention and progress of the sessions. Plan information usually includes:

- Frequency of appointments
- Continuation of step-by-step process as it unfolds session by session to achieve treatment plan goals
- Client self-care
- Referrals

Provide instruction for charting using either the textbook forms or modifications necessary for school charting forms.

MULTIPLE-CHOICE TEST BANK

_____ 1. Word elements:
   a. Have no meaning alone
   b. Can have prefixes substituted but not suffixes
   c. Include prefixes, root words, and suffixes
   d. Cannot be combined and make sense

_____ 2. The study of anatomy and physiology:
   a. Is needed only for working with sick people
   b. Is necessary to be able to understand massage benefits
   c. Should be kept separate from massage
   d. Provides information about function but not structure

_____ 3. A movement that increases the angle of a joint is:
   a. Adduction
   b. Extension
   c. Abduction
   d. Flexion

_____ 4. An agonist:
   a. Is responsible for primary movements
   b. Is a painful muscle
   c. Causes the relaxation response in a muscle
   d. Is a muscle that does not work in coordination with other muscles

_____ 5. An indication is when:
   a. An approach is contraindicated
   b. Cautions exist
   c. Massage should be avoided
   d. An approach would be beneficial

_____ 6. Goals for the massage session need to be:
   a. Quantified and qualified
   b. Based on massage experience
   c. Recorded on the physical assessment form
   d. Determined by the massage professional for the client

_____ 7. The information collected from the client during history taking and assessment procedures is called:
   a. A treatment plan
   b. Charting
   c. A database
   d. SOAP

_____ 8. Analysis process of the database includes:
   a. Review of the facts, generating possibilities and any impact on people involved
   b. Generating possibilities, pros and cons of each possibility, and any impact on people involved
   c. Review of the facts, generating possibilities, pros and cons of each possibility, and any impact on people involved
   d. Review of the facts, generating possibilities, and pros and cons of each possibility

_____ 9. A care of treatment plan is:
   a. Completed before data collection
   b. A guide to data analysis
   c. Not needed when working with pleasure goals
   d. A guide to reach agreed-on goals

_____ 10. SOAP is one type of:
   a. Assessment form
   b. Problem-oriented medical record
   c. Informed consent process
   d. Treatment plan development

_____ 11. A database consists of:
   a. Charts on the actual session
   b. All of the information available that contributes to therapeutic interaction
   c. The client's description of their problem
   d. Goals that are quantified and qualified, as well as functionally oriented.

_____ 12. The purpose of assessment is to:
   a. Provide methods to correct deviations from the norm
   b. Identify effective functioning so as to eliminate massage to that area
   c. Perform a visual and function assessment but not palpation assessment
   d. Identify effective functioning and deviations from the norm

_____ 13. A client presents a referral from his or her physician stating that only general massage with light pressure is to be used because of a recent angioplasty. The suffix in angioplasty means:
   a. Tumor
   b. Enlargement
   c. Surgical repair
   d. Disease

_____ 14. Record keeping for clients involves the following:
   a. Charting each session of the ongoing process
   b. Having the client fill out a general information packet
   c. Written record of intake procedures, informed consent, needs assessments, recording each session, and release of information
   d. Filing each piece of information received from physicians, insurance companies, or payments received from clients

The Scientific Art of Therapeutic Massage

▼INSTRUCTOROBJECTIVES

1. Cite current research that validates therapeutic massage.
2. Classify massage methods into basic concepts.
3. Explain the effects of therapeutic massage in physiologic terms.
4. Identify and categorize massage methods as reflexive or mechanical.

5. Explain anatomic and physiologic influences of massage on the neuroendocrine system, connective tissues, body circulation, and energy systems.
6. **Optional** Review stress management and the physiologic and psychologic aspects as discussed in Chapter 2, Mechanisms of Health and Disease, in *Mosby's Essential Sciences for Therapeutic Massage: Anatomy, Physiology, Biomechanics, and Pathology,* second edition.
7. **Optional** Define the parts and information of the nervous system in Chapters 4 and 5 in *Mosby's Essential Sciences.*

CHAPTER SUMMARY

The focus of this chapter is to establish an understanding of how massage affects physiology. The information presented is based on research related to the concept of why massage works. The scientific foundation for massage can then be expanded into artistic expression as massage methods are used to create the massage experience.

CHAPTER HIGHLIGHTS AND POINTS FOR DISCUSSION

The scientific approach to understanding anything involves observation, measurement of that which can be tested, accumulation of data, and analysis of the findings. Discuss the pros and cons of the scientific method.

Intuition is defined as knowing something without going through a conscious process of thinking. Other words for intuition include feelings, inspiration, instinct, revelation, impulse, and idea. Intuition is the ability to act purposefully on subconsciously perceived information. *Centering* is the ability to pay attention to, or focus on, a specific area. Centering skills allow us to screen sensation and concentrate. When we are centered, intuition is more apparent.

Art is defined as craft, skill, technique, and talent.

Discuss the role of intuition and art in the professional practice of therapeutic massage.

Although intuition and art are important, validating massage scientifically is equally important so as to separate what science knows and what is speculated about massage and related bodywork methods.

Discuss the pros and cons of speculation in terms of massage benefit.

Effective bodywork is achieved through the interaction of massage methods and physiology. Because this interaction occurs, the effects of massage can be studied through the scientific method. The scientific method is a way of *objectively* researching a concept to determine its validity. Research begins with a *hypothesis* or a statement expressed as, "If this happens, then that will happen." Next, the hypothesis is tested, usually with an *experiment.* The experiment needs to follow accepted design measures so that other researchers can replicate or redo the experiment. Results of the experiment will either prove or disprove the hypothesis. The results of the research often generate more questions that lead to more research.

Many exciting, ongoing massage-related studies are currently being conducted. The Touch Research Institute's more than 60 published and ongoing studies cover a broad range of subjects and conditions showing that massage affects many aspects of the human physiology and experience. Many other universities, medical schools, and research facilities are conducting research, and current research is being funded by the National Institutes of Health. Ongoing research in Europe and Asia will add to the validation of massage as a therapeutic intervention.

Discuss current research.

The manual techniques of massage are physiologically specific and well defined by the mode of application (i.e., rubbing, pulling, pressing, touching), the speed and depth of pressure (i.e., sustained or slow, rhythmic, staccato, or fast; light touch, deep touch, a combination of both), and the part of the therapist's body used to apply the techniques (i.e., fingers, hand, forearm, knee). The techniques of therapeutic massage and other types and styles of bodywork are merely variations of the fundamental application of manual manipulations providing external sensory stimulation. The effectiveness of the techniques is a result of basic physiologic effects.

Basic Physiologic Effects

1. Reflexive methods—physiologic responses are a result of homeostatic feedback loops (stimulus).
2. Mechanical methods—physiologic responses are a result of direct applications of methods (forces).

The problem with this simple categorization is that the mechanism by which the effects from massage are produced cannot always be clearly identified. To understand the basis of research findings, the practitioner must understand the mechanisms through which massage applications bring about the benefits indicated in the research. The areas of anatomic and physiologic influences are:

- Neuroendocrine system: central, autonomic, somatic nervous systems; neurochemicals; and hormones
- Connective tissues
- Circulations
- Energy systems

Discuss the physiologic interaction of massage applications in terms of how reflexive and mechanical stimulation of the body by massage might be beneficial. Following are guidelines for this discussion.

Effects of Massage on the Nervous System

Responses and effects of massage on the nervous system are primarily reflexive.

The nervous system responds to therapeutic massage methods through stimulation of sensory receptors. The sensory stimulation from massage disrupts an existing pattern in the central nervous system control centers, resulting in a shift of motor impulses, most often in the peripheral nervous system, which reestablishes homeostasis (Figure 4-1 in the textbook). Usually, both portions of the peripheral nervous system, somatic and autonomic, are influenced as balance is restored.

Neuroendocrine Interactions

The endocrine system is regulated through the influence of the nervous system, and the endocrine system, in turn, influences the nervous system. These two systems produce a large feedback loop similar to a thermostat on a furnace. The feedback system and autoregulation (maintenance of internal homeostasis) is linked with all body functions. The neurotransmitters and hormones carry messages that regulate physiologic functions. Research indicates that most behavior, mood, perceptions of stress and pain, and other so-called mental and emotional disorders are caused by either disregulation or failure of the biochemicals.

Influence of Massage on Neuroendocrine Substances

Some of the main neuroendocrine chemicals influenced by massage are:
- Dopamine
- Serotonin
- Epinephrine and adrenaline
- Norepinephrine and noradrenaline
- Enkephalins and endorphins
- Oxytocin
- Cortisol
- Growth hormone

Massage seems to increase available levels of dopamine and serotonin.

Massage seems to have a regulating effect on epinephrine and norepinephrine through either stimulating or inhibiting the sympathetic nervous system or stimulating or inhibiting the parasympathetic nervous system. This generalized balancing function of massage seems to recalibrate the appropriate adrenaline and noradrenaline levels.

Massage increases levels of enkephalins and endorphins.

Massage tends to increase levels of oxytocin. Oxytocin tends to increase feelings of connectedness, which might explain the connected and intimate feeling of massage.

Massage has been shown to reduce cortisol and substance P levels.

Massage increases availability of growth hormone indirectly by encouraging sleep and reducing cortisol levels.

Massage increases the blood levels of serotonin, dopamine, and endorphins, which, in turn, facilitate the production of natural killer cells in the immune system. This response indicates benefit in managing viral conditions and some forms of cancer as part of the total treatment program. At the same time, massage reduces cortisol and regulates epinephrine and norepinephrine, which facilitates the action of growth hormone.

Autonomic Influences

The effects of autonomic influences are primarily reflexive:
- Sympathetic activation and stress
- Parasympathetic patterns and conservation withdrawal
- Entrainment
- Body/mind effect
- Toughening/hardening
- Placebo effect

Sympathetic Activation and Stress

Studies involving slow-stroke back massage suggest a complex interaction among the autonomic, somatic, emotional, and cognitive elements in response to massage. All sensations, including touch, initially stimulate, whether they are received through visual, audio, or kinesthetic processes. Stimulation that is quick and unexpected will arouse. More commonly, massage encourages parasympathetic activation is encouraged by massage to counter the effects of sympathetic activation on arousal.

Entrainment

Entrainment is the coordination of, or synchronization to, a rhythm. Within the body, biologic oscillators such as the heart and thalamus seem to set the body's rhythm pattern. Body rhythms are also explained in *Mosby's Essential Sciences.*

To encourage entrainment, massage is provided in a quiet, rhythmic manner. The rhythmic application of massage and the proximity of a centered and compassionate professional's breathing rate, heart rate, and so forth can support restorative entrainment if body rhythms are not in synchronization. The focused and centered professional introduces his or her own ordered rhythms as part of the environment to add an additional external influence that enables the client's body rhythms to synchronize. When synchronization occurs, homeostatic mechanisms seem to operate more efficiently.

Body/Mind Effect

The body/mind link is best understood through the autonomic nervous system. An *altered state of consciousness* is any state of awareness that differs from the normal awareness of a conscious person. Altered states of consciousness are a factor in body/mind interactions.

Both the practitioner and the client can also achieve an altered state of consciousness during a bodywork session. When the altered state is achieved, it needs to be maintained for at least 15 minutes to best achieve therapeutic benefit.

State-Dependent Memory

Another aspect of the body/mind connection that interacts with the autonomic nervous system is state-dependent memory. Because of the effects of massage on the autonomic nervous system, massage can stimulate these state-dependent memory patterns.

Toughening/hardening is the reaction to repeated exposure to stimuli that elicit arousal responses. The planned presentation of stimuli teaches the body to manage more efficiently with sympathetic stress responses. Although massage is not as severe as cold shock, the increase in autonomic functioning and its passive nature may indeed be characterized as a form of passive toughening/hardening.

Influence of Massage on the Autonomic Nervous System

Because of its generalized effect on the autonomic nervous system and associated functions, massage can produce changes in mood and excitement levels and can induce the relaxation/restorative response. Massage seems to be a gentle modulator, producing feelings of general well being and comfort.

Additional information regarding the peripheral nervous system is located in *Mosby's Essential Sciences*, Chapter 5, "The Peripheral Nervous System. "

Somatic Influences

The effects of massage can be processed through the somatic division of the peripheral nervous system, which controls movement and muscle contraction/relaxation patterns, as well as muscle tone. Effects are primarily reflexive.

Somatic effects are produced through:
- Neuromuscular mechanisms
- Hyperstimulation analgesia
- Counterirritation
- Reduction of impingements (entrapment and compression)

Effect of Massage on the Somatic Nervous System

Massage methods directly stimulate the reflex mechanisms of the somatic functions. In fact, the bulk of the influence of massage is through somatic stimulation. The autonomic nervous system and endocrine system are often influenced by secondary reflex activity in response to homeostatic changes from somatic stimulation during massage. All massage methods are effective. The specific result depends on precise communication with the somatic sensory receptor. Massage is a language of pressure, pull, and movement.

Circulation

Circulation can be divided into three to five basic types. All anatomy textbooks recognize arterial, venous, and lymphatic circulation. The other two types of circulation are respiration and cerebral spinal fluid. These five systems are dependent on the pumping action of the skeletal muscles as they contract and relax. Arterial flow has additional pumping action provided by the heart and muscle tissue in the arteries. Research indicates that the lymphatic system has its own intrinsic rhythmic pump action. Some of the benefits of massage may be the result of the influence on this rhythm. These circulatory functions are directly linked, as well as interdependent. For example, the carbon dioxide levels of cerebral spinal fluid affect the respiratory center in the medulla, which helps control breathing.

Increases in the blood and lymph circulation are the most widely recognized physiologic effects of massage therapy.

How Massage Affects Circulation

Increased blood flow on a local level is achieved by compressing tissues, which empties venous beds, lowers venous pressure, and increases capillary blood flow, which is quickly counteracted by autoregulation. Massage stimulates the release of vasodilators, especially histamine. Blood flow changes may also be induced through the autonomic vascular reflexes. This particular increase in blood flow has a body-wide effect. Compression against arteries will mechanically influence the internal pressure receptors in the arteries. To avoid affecting the blood and lymph circulation while giving a massage seems impossible. Massage and other forms of bodywork mimic and assist the pumping action of the muscle and respiratory pump.

All massage approaches that restore mobility to the thorax and muscles of respiration affect the ability to breathe. Particularly with the breathing pattern disorder, retraining breathing is often ineffective because the mobility of the respiratory mechanism is disrupted. Massage is often able to restore the normal function of the soft tissue involved with breathing, allowing breathing retraining programs to become effective. Respiration, external and internal, is reviewed in *Mosby's Essential Sciences*.

Cerebral spinal fluid cools, nourishes, and influences breathing through carbon dioxide levels and protects the brain and nerves. The movement of this fluid has a pumping rhythm that can be palpated. This rhythm seems to affect the phenomenon of fascial movement and is independent of other body rhythms. Entrainment is implicated in fascial movement. More research needs to be done before the anatomic and physiologic mechanisms of the fascial movement phenomenon are scientifically understood. Techniques of cranial sacral therapy specifically affect cerebrospinal fluid circulation. General massage may also indirectly influence this mechanism. A more scientific explanation can be found in *Mosby's Essential Sciences*.

Connective Tissues

Connective tissue is the most abundant body tissue and is the structural component of the body. Functions of connective tissue include support, structure, space, stabilization, and scar formation. Connective tissue is made up of various fibers and cells in a gelatinous ground substance.

NOTE: *Mosby's Essential Sciences* **explains connective tissue and the different cell types.**

Healing of damage to body tissues requires the formation of connective tissue. The inflammatory response is one trigger that generates the healing process.

Piezoelectricity is an electric current produced by applying pressure to certain crystals such as mica, quartz, or Rochelle salt. Collagen seems to have a piezoelectric property. The piezoelectric phenomenon in some way affects the connective tissue properties. With its piezoelectric properties, the collagen portion of connective tissue may be the link to energy-related forms of bodywork.

Connective tissue methods are primarily mechanical. Connective tissue methods affect primarily the body structure. Methods that directly address the connective tissue do so by mechanically changing the consistency and pliability of the connective tissue, usually by softening it, and by creating physical space in the body. Bodywork methods most often affect the fascial sheaths (superficial and deep), ligaments, and tendons.

Two basic connective tissue methods are:
- Methods that address the *ground substance*. The ground substance is thrixtropic; that is, the substance liquifies on agitation and reverts to gel when standing. Ground substance is also a colloid. A colloid is a system of solids in a liquid medium that can resist abrupt pressure but yields to slow sustained pressure.
- Methods that address the *fibers* contained within the ground substance. The fibers are collagenous (ropes), elastic (rubber bands), or reticular (mesh).
- Methods that primarily affect the ground substance have a quality of slow, sustained pressure and agitation. Most massage methods can soften the ground substance, as long as the application is not abrupt.

The fiber component is affected by methods that elongate the fibers past the normal give or elastic range of the fiber and that enter the plastic range past the bind or point of restriction. This action creates either a freeing and unraveling of fibers or a small therapeutic (beneficial and controlled) inflammatory response that signals for change in the fibers. Transverse friction (see Chapter 11) also creates *therapeutic inflammation*.

Massage that provides for a gentle, sustained pull on the fascial component stimulates cutaneovisceral (skin to organ) reflex and, together with autonomic reflex pathways and endocrine response, produces the body-wide reactions to connective tissue massage.

Energy Systems

Both styles of massage (mechanical and reflexive) influence the energy component of the body by stimulating both electrical chemical and electrical magnetic effects. Scientific technology is beginning to allow measurement of this subtle component of the body. Consequently, the validity of the effectiveness of any modality that is based on the reaction of the electrical chemical or electrical magnetic component of the body is questionable. The term *subtle energies* or *biofield therapies* covers a wide range of techniques that affect the subtle electrical fields of the body. These electrical fields do exist. Animal behavior studies have shown that the platypus detects a living food source by sensing the weak electrical field around its prey. *Mosby's Essential Sciences*, Chapter 1, touches on electrical stimulation on and energy components within various sections throughout the chapter.

Effect of Massage on Body Energy

Sufficient research exists to demonstrate that modalities using *energy* have an effect through autonomic nervous system activity and endocrine responses in regard to entrainment, motor nerve points, and the piezoelectric properties of connective tissue fibers. Acupuncture points and meridians can be correlated directly to the nerve tracts and motor nerve points; chakras are located over nerve plexuses and biologic oscillators.

The interrelationship among all the body systems is sufficient to cause the body to respond to the stimulation of the innate electrical chemical energy with massage approaches. Therapeutic massage stimulates the nervous system and applies pressure on the connective tissues to produce a measurable electrical current via the piezoelectric properties of the connective tissue. The generalized therapeutic approach of massage seems to have a normalizing effect on the body's energetic processes.

MULTIPLE-CHOICE TEST BANK

_____ 1. Intuition:
   a. Is a sensation that cannot be defined
   b. Is knowing something without going through a rational thinking process
   c. Is an ability that cannot be defined
   d. Is not compatible with the scientific method

_____ 2. Given that massage affects physiology, it:
   a. Is not influenced by intuition
   b. Cannot be validated with the scientific method
   c. Can be studied by the scientific method
   d. Can be replaced by machine applications

_____ 3. Responses and effects of massage on the nervous system:
   a. Are mechanical
   b. Are not specific
   c. Are negligible
   d. Are reflexive

_____ 4. Neuroendocrine chemicals influenced by massage include:
   a. Dopamine and serotonin
   b. Cortisol and epidermis
   c. Plasma and parasympathetic
   d. Oxytocin and pacinian

_____ 5. Much of the body/mind connection takes place:
   a. Through somatic nervous system activity
   b. Through autonomic nervous system activity
   c. Through proprioceptors
   d. As a result of the general adaptation syndrome

_____ 6. Entrainment:
   a. Is synchronization to a rhythm
   b. Is seldom influenced by massage
   c. Is independent of external influences
   d. Has little effect on homeostasis

_____ 7. Entrapment:
   a. Does not occur at major nerve plexuses
   b. Will cause muscle pain but not breathing difficulties
   c. Interrupts the pain-spasm-pain cycle and initiates relaxation
   d. Is frequently caused by soft-tissue binding a nerve

_____ 8. Excessive prolonged stress:
   a. Will stop the parasympathetic response from occurring
   b. Is contraindicated for hyperstimulation analgesia
   c. Causes the release of cortisol
   d. Supports immune function

_____ 9. The two aspects of connective tissue most affected by massage are:
   a. Thrixtropic and cutaneovisceral
   b. Ground substance and fibers
   c. Plastic range and Meissner's corpuscles
   d. Piezoelectric and Merkel's disks

_____ 10. One of the most widely recognized physiologic effects of massage is:
   a. Compression
   b. An increase in fascial adhesions
   c. Enhancement in blood and lymph circulation
   d. Myofascial trigger points

_____ 11. Massage can increase a person's fine movement such as handwriting. Which neurotransmitter is influenced?
   a. Serotonin
   b. Oxytocin
   c. Dopamine
   d. Growth hormone

_____ 12. Parasympathetic patterns are:
- a. Restorative—adrenaline is secreted, mobility is decreased, and the bronchioles are constricted.
- **b. Physical activity is curtailed, digestion and elimination are increased, and the bronchioles are constricted.**
- c. Physical activity is increased, pupils are dilated, saliva secretion is stopped, and stomach secretion is increased.
- d. Restorative—heartbeat accelerates, bladder delays emptying, and saliva secretion is increased.

_____ 13. In the human body, what initiates entrainment?
- a. Digestive glands
- b. Autonomic nerves
- c. Brain
- **d. Biologic oscillators**

_____ 14. Your client gets a cramp in the hamstring when she stretches to quickly. Which reflex prompted the action?
- **a. Stretch reflex**
- b. Hooke's reflex
- c. Flexor reflex
- d. Extensor reflex

_____ 15. What is the best way to increase arterial flow circulation enhancement during massage?
- a. A 50-minute massage using effleurage but not heavy pressure
- **b. A 45-minute compressive massage against the arteries proximal to the heart and moving in a distal direction**
- c. A 50-minute massage using short pumping effleurage and gliding toward the heart
- d. Receive a massage for 30 minutes, emphasizing gliding strokes to passive/active joint movement from distal to proximal

Indications and Contraindications for Therapeutic Massage

▼ CONTENT OUTLINE

▼ INSTRUCTOR OBJECTIVES

1. Define indication and contraindication.
2. Present indications for massage therapy and justify these indications.

NOTE: **Use the pathology appendix in *Mosby's Essential Sciences for Therapeutic Massage: Anatomy, Physiology, Biomechanics, and Pathology,* second edition, text and the indications and contraindications located at the end of each chapter section. Also, Chapter 15 in this text has case studies that can be referred to as necessary.**

3. Explain the difference between objective and subjective massage benefits.
4. Define therapeutic change, condition management, and palliative care.
5. Explain the concepts of therapeutic change, condition management, and palliative care in relation to indications and contraindications for massage.
6. Reinforce the clinical reasoning process to assist the student in making the appropriate decisions regarding the type of care that is most beneficial for the client.
7. Present a basic understanding of pathology and its connection to contraindications to massage. A Pathology Appendix in *Mosby's Essential Sciences* is an excellent reference for this objective.

8. Present criteria to evaluate a client's status to determine if massage is contraindicated.
9. Define health, dysfunction, and pathology.
10. Present criteria to help a student recognize when a primary health care provider should evaluate a client's condition.
11. Discuss the mechanisms and risk factors that predispose people to disease processes.
12. Present the warning signs of cancer.
13. Explain the general inflammatory response.
14. Explain the mechanisms of pain and evaluate pain for referral purposes. Chapter 2 in *Mosby's Essential Sciences* reviews pain and the various types of pain.
15. Present the endangerment sites for massage.
16. Explain methods for referring a client to a primary health care provider.
17. Provide guidelines for interpreting the reference list of indications and contraindications provided in Appendix A and medications in Appendix C.

CHAPTER SUMMARY

The massage professional must be able to identify indications and contraindications for therapeutic massage. This chapter provides the information necessary to make important decisions regarding the application of massage based on the benefits that therapeutic massage provides. Also explored are various approaches to care based on the client's condition and realistic goals that may be achieved through using therapeutic massage. Contraindications are also presented along with guidelines for decision making with regard to the type of contraindications and whether massage should be avoided, should be modified, or is applicable only with appropriate supervision. Case studies that model the decision-making process are presented.

CHAPTER HIGHLIGHTS AND POINTS FOR DISCUSSION

An *indication* tells when an approach would be beneficial for health enhancement, for treating a particular condition, or to support a treatment modality other than massage.
A *contraindication* tells when an approach might be harmful. Types of contraindications are:
1. General avoidance of application—do not massage.
2. Regional avoidance of application—massage is permitted, but avoid a particular area.
3. Application with caution, usually requiring supervision from appropriate medical or supervising personnel—massage is permitted, but carefully select the type of methods to be used, the duration of the massage, and the frequency.

Discuss criteria that would help categorize the three types of contraindications.

Indications for massage are based on the health-enhancing benefits of massage. The benefits of massage therapy are both objective and subjective. That is, some results of massage can be measured (objective), whereas others are only assumed to be effective based on experience (subjective).

Discuss the difference between subjective and objective benefits.

The benefits of massage occur as a result of therapeutic change, condition management, and palliative care.

Any change process, including beneficial change, requires energy and resource expenditure by the client. Decisions need to be made about the ability of the client to expend the energy required for active change and about the availability of the support and resources that are often necessary during a change process. The practitioner requires appropriate knowledge and skills (current or acquired) and often a network of support from other professionals to facilitate a change process.

Discuss why the change process is dependent on energy expenditure.

Condition management involves using massage methods to support the clients who are unable to undergo a therapeutic change process but wish to be as effective as possible within an existing set of circumstances. On a physical level, massage can offer benefit by managing the existing physical compensation patterns and sometimes slowing the progress of the chronic conditions or preventing a situation from becoming worse. On an emotional level, massage can assist in managing physical stress symptoms to allow the person to better cope with the life stresses that cannot be altered. Condition management accounts for the largest client base for therapeutic massage.

Discuss why condition management is the largest client base for therapeutic massage.

To *palliate* is to soothe or relieve. Massage is soothing and provides comfort regardless of whether the client is seeking relaxation to meet pleasure needs or to cope with chronic pain. In a health care context, the term *palliative care* means to relieve or reduce the intensity of uncomfortable symptoms but not to produce a cure.

Palliative care is provided when the condition is most likely going to become worse and when degenerative processes will continue, as in terminal illness or dementia. Palliative care often relates to approaches that reduce suffering.

Palliative care is also appropriate when the condition should not be changed or the person does not desire a specific outcome other than pleasure and relaxation.

Discuss the importance of pleasure and relaxation as outcomes.

Massage professionals need to understand basic pathology. Although the diagnosis of disorders is not a function of a massage professional, to refer appropriately, the massage professional must be able to recognize when the client's condition represents an irregularity that should be evaluated by his or her primary health care provider. When working with a referral and under proper supervision, the massage professional also needs to be able to alter the application of massage in terms of any present disease process such that the client receives the benefits of massage without harm. The massage professional also needs a basic understanding of pharmacology and the possible interactions between medications and massage. See Appendix C for specific information.

Discuss indications for referral and health care supervision. Also discuss other forms of supervision in different environments such as the athletic trainer when working with athletes.

Health is defined as optimal functioning with freedom from disease or abnormal processes. Health is influenced by many factors, including inherited (genetic) and constitutional conditions. Lifestyle, activity, level, rest, loving relationships, exercise, a balanced diet, empowering beliefs and attitudes, self-esteem, authentic personality, and freedom from self-hindering patterns all support health. Mechanisms of health can also be found in *Mosby's Essential Sciences* for an additional source.

Dysfunction is the in-between state of *not healthy* but also *not sick* (experiencing disease). Western medicine has difficulty identifying and dealing with dysfunctions because they are prepathologic states and are often not apparent within current diagnostic methods. Prevention methods, many modeled after more *Eastern* or *holistic approaches,* are beginning to address this area called dysfunction.

Disease or *pathologic conditions* occur when homeostatic and restorative body mechanisms break down and can no longer adapt. Seldom does one thing contribute to disease; instead a series of events occurs.

The body has anatomic and physiologic functioning limits. Extraordinary events push the body's limits of functioning. Normal physiologic mechanisms inhibit the tendency to function at body limits. Dysfunction occurs when the reserve runs low because restorative mechanisms are not able to function effectively or when the body begins to limit function in an attempt to maintain higher energy reserves.

Massage professionals serve many people at the beginning of dysfunctional patterns, when clients do not feel their best but are not yet sick. The practitioner must monitor clients to make sure they do not continue to progress further into dysfunctional patterns. Early intervention and referral to the appropriate health care professional are important to identify potential problems before they develop. The benefits of massage are most effectively focused when they help people stay within the healthy range of functioning.

Discuss the different applications of massage for health maintenance, dysfunction, and disease or pathologic condition.

Because most diseases have similar symptoms, determining the specific underlying causes of disease is difficult. Disease conditions are usually diagnosed or identified by signs and symptoms. Certain predisposing conditions may make developing a disease more likely. Usually called *risk factors,* these conditions may put an individual at risk for developing a disease but often do not actually cause the disease.

Discuss various risk factors.

The *general adaptation syndrome* describes how the body mobilizes different defense mechanisms when threatened by harmful (actual or perceived) stimuli.

Discuss the general adaptation syndrome and its relationship to health and disease.

Inflammation may occur as a response to any tissue injury. Local inflammation occurs in a limited area, for example, a small cut that becomes infected. Systemic inflammation occurs when the irritant spreads throughout the body or when inflammation mediators cause changes throughout the body. Conditions involving chronic inflammation are classified as inflammatory diseases. Therapeutic massage seems to be beneficial in cases of prolonged inflammation.

The processes of inflammation trigger tissue repair. A goal in the healing process is to promote regeneration and minimize replacement. Massage has been shown to slow the formation of scar tissue and keep scar tissue pliable when it forms.

Therapeutic Inflammation

Because the inflammatory response is part of a healing process, the deliberate creation of inflammation can generate or "jump start" healing mechanisms. Certain methods of massage can be used to create a controlled, localized area of therapeutic inflammation. The benefit derived from using therapeutic inflammation depends on the body's ability to generate a healing process. If healing mechanisms are suppressed, do not use methods that create therapeutic inflammation. Therapeutic inflammation is not used in situations in which disturbed sleep, compromised immune function, a high degree of stress load, or systemic or localized inflammation is already present. These methods should also be avoided if any condition such as fibromyalgia exists, which consists of impaired repair and restorative functions, unless carefully supervised as part of a total treatment program.

Consideration needs to be given to using antiinflammatory medications. If a person is using such a medication, either steroidal or nonsteroidal, the effectiveness of therapeutic inflammation is negated or reduced, and restoration mechanisms are inhibited. When these medications are present, any methods that create inflammation should be avoided.

Discuss the indications and contraindications, including cautions, for using therapeutic inflammation.

Pain

The massage therapist especially needs to understand the mechanisms of pain. The main types of pain are:
- Acute
- Chronic
- Intractable
- Phantom

Pain has many characteristics. Location of pain can be divided into four categories:
- Localized pain is pain confined to the site of origin.
- Projected pain is typically a result of proximal nerve compression. This pain is perceived in the tissue supplied by the nerve.
- Radiating pain is diffuse pain around the site of origin that is not well localized.
- Referred pain is felt in an area distant from the site of the painful stimulus.

Five types of pain experience include the following:
- Pricking or bright pain
- Burning pain
- Aching pain
- Deep pain
- Muscle pain

The origins of pain can be divided into two types, somatic and visceral.

The ability of the cerebral cortex to locate the origin of pain is related to experience. In most instances of somatic pain, and in some instances of visceral pain, the cortex accurately projects the pain back to the stimulated area.

In general, the area to which the pain is referred and the visceral organ involved receive their innervation from the same segment of the spinal cord. As already stated, irritation of the viscera frequently produces pain that is felt not in the viscera but in some somatic structure that may be located at a considerable distance.

Pain is a complex problem with physical, psychologic, social, and financial components. Pain can be alleviated in many ways. The massage professional, as part of a health care team, can contribute valuable manual therapy in various pain conditions using direct tissue manipulation and reflex stimulation of the nervous system and circulation. As a therapeutic intervention, massage may help reduce the need for pain medication, thus reducing the side effects of medication use. Intervention for acute pain is less invasive and more focused on supporting a current healing process. Chronic pain is managed with either symptom relief or a more aggressive rehabilitation approach incorporating a therapeutic change process.

Discuss pain origin. Also discuss the difference in massage for acute pain and chronic pain. Discuss mechanisms stimulated by massage that reduce pain perception, including gait control, counterirritation, hyperstimulation, analgesia, and changes in neurotransmitters and hormones.

Nerve Impingement

The two types of nerve impingement are compression and entrapment. Massage is beneficial for entrapment and can manage some symptoms of nerve compression, even though the direct causal factor is not addressed. Massage methods can soften and stretch connective tissues that may impinge on nerves, as well as normalize muscle tension patterns, restoring a more normal resting length to short muscles to reduce pressure on nerves.

Discuss the difference between impingement and compression syndromes.

Psychologic Effects

Science has validated the body/mind link in terms of heath and disease. Many risk factors for developing physical (body) disease are mentally (mind) influenced, such as stress level and lifestyle choices. The major mental heath dysfunctions affecting Western society are trauma and posttraumatic stress disorders, anxiety and depression, pain and fatigue syndromes often coupled with anxiety and depression, and stress-related illness.

Because massage intervention has a strong physiologic effect resulting from the comfort of compassionate touch, as well as an influence on mental state through the effect on the autonomic nervous system and neurochemicals, massage may be beneficial for individuals experiencing mental health problems. Managing pain is an important intervention. Because therapeutic massage can often offer symptomatic relief from chronic pain, the feelings of helplessness that accompany these difficulties may dissipate as the person realizes that management methods are available. Soothing of any hyperactivity or hypoactivity of the autonomic nervous system provides a sense of inner balance. Normalizing the breathing mechanism allows a person to breathe without restriction and can reduce the tendency toward breathing pattern disorder, which feeds anxiety and panic.

Strong and appropriate indications exist for using massage therapy in restoring mental health, but caution is indicated in terms of establishing dual roles and boundary difficulties. Working in conjunction with mental health providers in these situations is important.

Discuss the body/mind influence on health. Discuss the benefits of massage intervention for mental health. Discuss breathing pattern disorder and the link between mental and physical interactions.

Contraindications

A contraindication is any condition that renders a particular treatment improper or undesirable, or when cautions concerning treatment exist and supervision is required.

Contraindications can be separated into three types: general, regional, and cautions.

Therapeutic massage is often beneficial for clients who are receiving treatment for a specific medical or mental health condition, but *caution is indicated*. The general effects of stress and pain reduction, increased circulation, and physical comfort of therapeutic massage complement most other medical and mental health treatment modalities. However, when other therapies, including medication, are being used, the physician must be able to evaluate accurately the effectiveness of each treatment the client is receiving. If the physician is not aware that the client is receiving massage, the effects of other therapies may be misinterpreted.

Immediately refer patients with any vague or unexplainable symptoms of fatigue, muscle weakness, and general aches and pains to a physician. Many disease processes share these symptoms.

Massage is not necessarily contraindicated for individuals with cancer. Current research indicates that massage can support the immune system battle with cancer cells. However, massage must be used as part of the entire treatment program and supervised by qualified medical personnel. As with any stressful condition, when working with people with cancer, it is important not to overtax their system, but to instead use massage for a general support to the healing mechanisms of the body.

Discuss various contraindications and factors that influence how to determine whether massage is appropriate. Discuss how interventions that might be contraindicated without medical supervision might be appropriate with proper supervision.

The massage professional needs to be aware of the client's medications. In general, a medication is prescribed to do one of the following:

• Stimulate a body process
• Inhibit a body process
• Replace a chemical in the body

Therapeutic massage can also stimulate, inhibit, and replace body functions. When the medication and massage both stimulate the same process, the effects are synergistic, and the result can be too much stimulation. If the medication inhibits a process and massage inhibits the same process, the result is again synergistic, but this time with too much inhibition. If the medication stimulates an effect and massage inhibits the same effect, massage can be antagonistic to the medication. Although massage seldom interacts substantially with medications that replace a body chemical, the massage practitioner must be aware of possible synergistic or inhibitory effects.

Massage can often be used to manage undesirable side effects of medications. Be aware of any over-the-counter medications, herbs, and vitamins that the patient may be taking as well. If a client is taking medication, the physician must be contacted for recommendations about the advisability of therapeutic massage.

Discuss various classifications of medication. See Appendix C in the textbook.

Endangerment sites are areas in which nerves and blood vessels surface close to the skin and are not well protected by muscle or connective tissue. Consequently, deep sustained pressure into these areas might damage the vessels and nerves. Areas where fragile bony projections might be broken off are also considered endangerment sites. The kidney area is included as such a site because the kidneys are loosely suspended in fat and connective tissue. Heavy pounding is contraindicated in that area. Avoidance or light pressure is indicated if working over an endangerment site to avoid any damage to the area.

Discuss and identify the location of various endangerment sites.

Referral is a method by which a client is sent to a health care professional for diagnosis and treatment of a disease.

Discuss indications and methods for referral.

MULTIPLE-CHOICE TEST BANK

_____ 1. The implementation of a therapeutic change process requires:
   a. Maintaining the current condition with less suffering
   b. Energy and resource expenditure
   c. Continued deterioration of client's symptoms
   d. Weekly sessions for an extended period

_____ 2. The body/mind link is best understood:
   a. As having no physiologic basis
   b. Through cerebral spinal fluid movement
   c. As separate from hormone interplay
   d. In autonomic nervous system association

_____ 3. The benefits of massage:
   a. Can be subjective and objective
   b. Are entirely subjective
   c. Have little supportive research
   d. Are entirely biomechanic

_____ 4. Which of the following statements is true?
   a. Massage does not significantly affect physiologic function.
   b. The underlying causes of disease are easy to determine.
   c. Massage professionals need to know about pathology.
   d. Always believe clients if they say that their health is excellent.

_____ 5. Which of the following is NOT a major risk factor?
   a. Syndrome
   b. Age
   c. Lifestyle
   d. Environment

_____ 6. The general adaptation syndrome was described by:
   a. Hans Tagether
   b. Tiffany Field
   c. John Yates
   d. Hans Selye

_____ 7. With regard to pain sensation:
   a. Pain receptors adapt easily.
   b. Nociceptors are the hormones that result from pain.
   c. Hyperalgesia is the normal response to gentle touch.
   d. It is classified as acute, chronic, or intractable.

_____ 8. Endangerment sites:
   a. Need deep sustained pressure to minimize damage
   b. Include the axillary and umbilicus area
   c. Include the second and third ribs
   d. Refer to organ reflexes, not nerve and blood vessels

_____ 9. Contraindications to massage include:
   a. Any condition that might render massage undesirable or improper
   b. Primarily avoidance of massage with few cautions
   c. Circulation enhancement, pain control, and musculoskeletal discomfort
   d. Any conditions that do not require analgesics

_____ 10. Which of the following is NOT necessarily a reason for referral?
   a. Bleeding and bruising
   b. Inflammation and fever
   c. Being overweight
   d. Lumps and tissue changes

_____ 11. Condition management involves using massage methods to support clients who cannot undergo a therapeutic change but wish to be as effective as possible within an existing set of circumstances. Which of the following is an example of condition management?
   a. Managing the existing physical compensation patterns
   b. Assisting the client in learning to walk again
   c. Restoring a client's range of motion to be injury state.
   d. Using massage to help a client feel better about self and change his or her job

_____ 12. Homeostasis can be defined as:
   a. The process of counterbalancing a defect in body structure or function
   b. A group of signs and symptoms
   c. The relative constancy of the body's internal environment
   d. The subjective abnormalities that a person feels

_____ 13. Massage has been shown to slow formation of scar tissue and helps keep scar tissue pliable. This result assists the healing process by:
   a. Blocking the action of antihistamines
   b. Counterbalancing the defect in the body
   c. Promoting regeneration and keeping replacement to a minimum
   d. Keeping the functioning energy reserves in place

_____ 14. Therapeutic inflammation can be accomplished most effectively through:
   a. Deep frictioning and connective tissue stretching
   b. Gliding
   c. Effleurage
   d. Tapotement and rapid compression

_____ 15. What is the process that occurs when medication and message both stimulate the same process?
   a. Antagonistic
   b. Synergistic
   c. Metastasis
   d. Impingement

CHAPTER 6

Hygiene, Sanitation, and Safety

▼CONTENT**OUTLINE**

▼INSTRUCTOR**OBJECTIVES**

1. Present good health and personal hygiene practices.
2. Explain the major disease-causing agents.
3. Present the transmission routes for disease-causing pathogens.
4. Describe methods for prevention and control of disease.
5. Demonstrate sanitation practices, including Standard Precautions, to prevent and control the spread of disease.
6. Give specific recommendations for sanitary practices for massage businesses.
7. Present how to implement Standard Precautions.
8. Provide information about human immunodeficiency virus (HIV), acquired immunodeficiency syndrome (AIDS), and hepatitis.
9. Identify behavior that is suspected to transmit HIV and hepatitis virus.
10. Develop criteria to enable the student to create a safe and hazard-free massage environment.
11. Complete an accident report.

CHAPTER SUMMARY

This chapter describes hygiene and sanitation practices in a professional setting. The massage professional must provide both a sanitary and safe environment. An important responsibility is to consider fire and accident prevention for both the client and the professional. The information presented may seem as common sense, but specific skills are required to practice massage in a way that protects the safety of both the client and the massage professional.

CHAPTER HIGHLIGHTS AND POINTS FOR DISCUSSION

The primary importance of sanitation is to prevent the spread of contagious disease. Diseases caused by "germs" or viruses, bacteria, fungi, and parasites are considered contagious. Contagious diseases are best controlled by using sanitary practices before infection results.

Because new information concerning the spread and control of contagious diseases is being dispersed almost daily, the practitioner must stay current. The Centers for Disease Control and Prevention (CDC) Standards and Guidelines for Communicable Diseases may change as new information becomes available. The massage practitioner must update information biannually regarding changes in CDC recommendations and follow the most current standards and guidelines.

Discuss contagious diseases in relation to sanitation. We must take care of ourselves not only so that we function at our best, but also because, as wellness and health professionals, we set an example for our clients. The following must be considered:

- Personal health
- Smoking
- Alcohol and drugs
- Hygiene

Discuss why the health and hygiene of the massage practitioner are important professional issues.

Sanitary massage methods promote conditions that are conducive to health, meaning that pathogenic organisms must be eliminated or controlled. Pathogens are spread by direct contact, through blood or other fluids, or by being airborne.

Pathogenic Organisms

Pathogenic organisms cause the development of many disease processes. These organisms include viruses, bacteria, fungi, protozoa, and pathogenic animals.

The key to preventing many diseases caused by pathogenic organisms is to stop the organisms from entering the human body. The following is a partial list of the ways in which pathogens can spread:

- Environmental contact
- Opportunistic invasion
- Person-to-person contact

Aseptic technique involves killing or disabling pathogens on surfaces before they can spread to people.

Most sanitation conditions for massage require disinfection. Protective apparel is occasionally necessary. In rare instances, using gloves, masks, and gowns may be appropriate to protect the massage professional or client.

Proper hand washing is the single most effective deterrent to the spread of disease.

Standard Precautions, issued in 1987 by the CDC and in 1989 by the Bureau of Communicable Disease and Epidemiology in Canada, prevent the spread of both bacterial and viral infections. Developed initially to prevent the spread of blood-borne diseases such as HIV and hepatitis B, Standard Precautions support a safe and sanitary environment. Guidelines for Standard Precautions include specific recommendations for using gloves, masks, and protective eyewear when contact with blood or body secretions is possible. Standard Precautions also include recommendations for clean-up procedures.

Standard Precautions prevent the spread of hepatitis. The massage practitioner must avoid all behaviors that are potential transmission routes for HIV and hepatitis B virus.

Discuss appropriate sanitation methods for the massage professional.

Most accidents can be prevented. Knowing the common safety hazards, recognizing which clients need extra assistance, and using common sense are all necessary to promote safety. When an accident occurs, an accident report is required.

Discuss how to create a safe environment for both the massage professional and massage clients.

MULTIPLE-CHOICE TEST BANK

_____ 1. Which of the following is not a method that spreads disease?
    a. Person-to-person contact
    b. Disinfection
    c. Opportunistic invasion
    d. Environmental contact

_____ 2. Suggested sanitation for all massage requirements include:
    a. Using gloves and masks
    b. Using sterilization procedures
    c. Using an antibacterial/antiviral cleaning agent
    d. Wearing protective apparel

_____ 3. While cleaning in the massage area:
    a. Store linens in a closed bag or container.
    b. Shake out all linens to remove dust.
    c. Work from the dirtiest area to the cleanest.
    d. Clean while moving dirt toward your body.

_____ 4. Standard Precautions:
    a. Should not be used by unlicensed massage therapists
    b. Have no application to massage
    c. Currently recommend using gloves for all massages
    d. Prevent the spread of infections

_____ 5. To clean spills of body fluids:
   a. Use a 10% bleach solution.
   b. Use hot water.
   c. Use diluted hydrogen peroxide.
   d. Use soap.

_____ 6. HIV is a virus:
   a. That is the only known deadly virus
   b. That lives in red blood cells
   c. That can be killed with hot soapy water and a 10% bleach solution
   d. That affects mainly the skin and hair

_____ 7. AIDS:
   a. Causes HIV
   b. Is thought to be caused by a bacteria
   c. Is caused by weak lymphocytes
   d. Is a dysfunction of the immune system

_____ 8. Viruses:
   a. Can be killed by antibiotics
   b. Can live in the body without causing any symptoms to appear
   c. Cannot live in mucous membrane
   d. Cannot infect healthy people

_____ 9. Hepatitis:
   a. Is a liver inflammation caused by a virus
   b. Is a blood inflammation caused by a bacteria
   c. Is not contagious
   d. Is not a contraindication for massage

_____ 10. To improve safety in the massage therapy environment:
   a. Regularly check and maintain all equipment and tables.
   b. Keep all electrical cords hidden under the rugs.
   c. Keep tile floors highly polished.
   d. Provide candles in case of power failure.

_____ 11. Pathogens are spread by three main routes. Which of the following is one of these routes?
   a. Opportunistic invasion
   b. Clean uniform
   c. Intact skin
   d. Aseptic technique

_____ 12. Pathogenic disease causing organisms include:
   a. Dirt, sweat, and grime
   b. Paint, tar, and dust
   c. Viruses, bacteria, and fungi
   d. Smoking, drinking, and washing

Body Mechanics

▼ INSTRUCTOR OBJECTIVES

1. Demonstrate the use of the body when giving a massage, especially the hands and forearms, in an efficient and biomechanically correct manner.
2. Describe and demonstrate how to alter position of both the client and the practitioner to maximize body mechanics.
3. Explain the importance of body mechanics and why continuing education regarding body mechanics is important after graduating.
4. Teach the student to self-assess body mechanics using the Rubric (see Appendix), and have the students use it as a reminder to correct improper body mechanics.

CHAPTER SUMMARY

This chapter presents the importance of proper use of the body while giving a massage. Body mechanics allow the massage practitioner's body to be used in a careful, efficient, and deliberate way. Body mechanics involve good posture, balance, leverage, and using the strongest and largest muscles to perform the work. In this chapter, the student will learn methods of working more efficiently so that providing 8 hours of massage in a day does not cause any dysfunction or pain.

SPECIAL NOTE TO INSTRUCTORS: This chapter is important. The illustrations are helpful, especially when used to position the students. The following drill is useful when teaching body mechanics:

1. Identify the "hill" on the body against which you want to lean.
2. Walk up to the table and place both thighs against the table in relation to the hill against which to be leaned so that the practitioner is placed near the bottom of the hill.
3. Raise the arm that points to the area against which to be leaned. Keep the arm parallel to the table.
4. Line up the crease of the elbow of the raised arm so that it is pointing to the area against which to be leaned. Move the entire body either left or right until the position is found.
5. Keep this arm out—this will be the weight-bearing arm. Do not put it down or you (the student) may become confused.
6. Place and maintain the feet shoulder-width apart—NOT like standing on a tight rope.
7. Depending on the depth of pressure, take a one fourth, one half, or full step back. The farther from the table you are standing, the more pressure will be delivered.

8. Pivot both feet so that the toes are pointing toward the area against which to be leaned. Do not pick the feet up from the floor—pivot on the balls of the foot. Turn both feet to make sure that the pelvis and shoulders are pointing in the same direction, and bring the knee into the proper position for weight bearing. Otherwise the pelvis is twisted, the knee cannot move into the knee-lock position, and weight bearing puts strain on the collateral ligaments.

9. Identify the back leg, which will be the weight-bearing leg. Maintain weight on the heel.

10. The front leg is used for stability and to transfer weight when moving; it should not bear weight and should be able to be raised off the floor.

11. Aim and fall gently forward from your belly to make contact with the practice client's body. The pressure comes from the weight-bearing leg, abdomen, and torso generated through the arm. The body leaned against should move down and forward in response to the pressure. If the practitioner's contact arm is pulled away, the practitioner should lose his or her balance.

12. Do not bend elbows, tense wrists, bend at the waist, or balance on the weight-bearing leg.

13. Do not permanently shift the weight to the front foot when moving to a different position on the client's body. When moving to a different position on the body, move the back foot behind the front foot and relean.

14. Do not attempt to apply pressure down a hill. If necessary, slide down the hill to get to the next hill before pressure bearing.

15. Shift foot position as indicated in step 14 when not bearing pressure.

NOTE: **Principles of biomechanics are explained in Chapter 10 of *Mosby's Essential Sciences for Therapeutic Massage: Anatomy, Physiology, Biomechanics, and Pathology*, second edition. The biomechanics presented in this text are based on these principles.**

This drill teaches the concept of leaning. After the student can lean effectively, teach how to use the front leg and opposite arm as stabilizers. Because students are often afraid of applying too much pressure, they avoid leaning to provide leverage for body mechanics. Instead, students push, using muscle strength to apply pressure. This approach often results in uneven pressure and a narrow point of distribution of the pressure, such as occurs when the tip of the elbow is used to apply pressure. The client experiences a "poking" sensation that is uncomfortable. In addition, using muscle strength is energy consuming and therefore fatiguing for the practitioner.

The instructor should have the student contrast the correct and incorrect methods. Have the student notice what happens when he or she shifts the weight to the front foot,

bends the elbow, or tightens the wrists, bends at the waist, and attempts to apply the same type of pressure. Have practice clients on the table supply feedback to the student.

The video available through Mosby that accompanies this chapter (*Mosby's Fundamentals of Therapeutic Massage Video Series*, video 1, "Massage Overview and Draping Procedures") is helpful when teaching these skills.

Position a practice client on the table and identify hills. Use supine, prone, side-lying, and seated positions; compare and contrast the advantages of each position in terms of body mechanics. Side-lying position often offers some of the best advantages for body mechanics and should be used more often for massage. This position offers easy access to the medial and lateral side of the leg in a position with hills that are available against which to be leaned. The lateral thorax is best accessed in this position, as is the neck, arm, and shoulder. The supine position offers the least mechanical advantage because few hills are available. Many students avoid the side-lying position because they are uncomfortable with draping and bolstering in this position. This avoidance is unfortunate because working in the most energy-conserving way while accomplishing the most benefit for the client is important. Draping is covered in the next chapter.

NOTE: **Asian form stances are ineffective as body mechanics when giving a massage because the focus of Asian disciplines is maintaining balance and dropping the center of gravity down between the feet. Transferring weight as used during massage is the opposite.**

CHAPTER HIGHLIGHTS AND POINTS FOR DISCUSSION

Delivery of therapeutic massage makes unique postural and physical demands. A majority of the effort exerted to give a massage is a sustained, restrained, and somewhat static movement, with pressure focused down to deliver compressive force.

Discuss how the delivery of compressive force is different from lifting. Areas of the body commonly affected in the massage professional who is not attentive to body mechanics include the neck and shoulder, wrist and thumb, lower back, knee, ankle, and foot.

Using the transfer of body weight and not muscle strength to provide the pressure required during a massage is vital. The amount of pressure to be applied is increased by widening the stance, which is accomplished by moving the back leg farther away from the point of contact, but do not stand on the toes. If heavy pressure is required, use the *lean and lift approach* described in the text to apply counter pressure.

Massage primarily uses a force generated forward and downward. Therefore redistributing the center of gravity and the weight force forward becomes necessary by keeping the weight on the back leg and the balance point at the object-contact point.

The arm generating the pressure is opposite of the weight-bearing leg, which allows proper counterbalance and prevents twisting of the body.

When the practitioner's weight is maintained on the back foot, the pressure levels are more even; but when the weight shifts to the front foot, the pressure becomes more concentrated, uneven, and pokey, and may be uncomfortable for the client.

The massage table must be at a comfortable height, which depends on the body size and style of the practitioner. If the massage professional is carrying a portable table, attention should be paid to the body mechanics used to lift and move the table. If the massage professional chooses to work on a mat on the floor, the same body mechanics principles apply. The balance points will then be from the knees instead of the feet.

The massage professional's body is an important tool that is not replaceable. Taking care of ourselves while giving a massage is critical. If the professional is uncomfortable, the client will become uncomfortable. If the massage practitioner can give a massage in a relaxed, efficient, and energy-conserving manner, the client will be able to relax and more easily accept the touch.

Discuss the importance of the efficient use of the practitioner's body as a tool. Discuss modification of body mechanics by demonstrating the use of a stool, chair, and so on.

Discuss and demonstrate the various principles of body mechanics presented in the text. Review this information during discussion of positioning and draping in Chapter 8.

Continue to reinforce the importance of body mechanics when teaching technical skills.

MULTIPLE-CHOICE TEST BANK

_____ 1. Proper application of body mechanics principles:
    a. Involves good posture and balance
    b. Involves the use of muscle strength to apply pressure
    c. Will prevent fatigue by not causing overuse syndromes
    d. Will be exactly the same for each individual

_____ 2. Areas of the massage professional's body commonly under stress include:
    a. Primarily the shoulder and the wrist
    b. The neck, shoulder, arm, hand, low back, and leg
    c. Only the hand and the knee
    d. Primarily the hand and the thumb

_____ 3. A massage therapist can prevent dysfunction by:
    a. Maintaining a 90-degree angle at the wrist during compression
    b. Standing still and limiting movement
    c. Working efficiently by using the body weight and not muscle strength
    d. Keeping both feet flat on the floor at all times

_____ 4. A general rule that applies to body mechanics is:
    a. Keep feet as close together as possible.
    b. Keep weight on the front foot.
    c. Stay ahead of the stroke.
    d. Keep wrists and hands relaxed.

_____ 5. The massage practitioner's knees:
    a. Should be in the normal screw home position while standing
    b. Need compressive forces increased
    c. Increase the joint capsule as they stabilize
    d. Have the least compressive force on the joint when flexed

_____ 6. Massage primarily uses a force generated:
    a. Forward and backward
    b. Forward and downward
    c. Upward and downward
    d. Backward and forward

_____ 7. The best way to use the body efficiently is to:
    a. Be cool, calm, and collected.
    b. Work hard, using compressive force.
    c. Stand straight and bend at the waist.
    d. Remain relaxed, comfortable, and do not strain.

_____ 8. Correct body mechanics include weight on the back foot with:
    a. The same-side working hand
    b. The opposite working hand
    c. The front foot placed firmly on the floor
    d. A position facing 90 degrees to the generated line of pressure

_____ 9. Triangles should be used:
   a. As guidelines to determine distance from the contact hand or forearm
   b. As a rule to determine knee angle
   c. To place on a short stool so it is the right height
   d. To help carry a portable table

_____ 10. Increase or decrease in the amount of pressure delivered is determined by:
   a. Symmetrical stance in the forward position
   b. Whether the hand or forearm is used
   c. Distance of the back foot from the massage table
   d. Asymmetric stance and feet placed shoulder width apart

_____ 11. When a practitioner is in a relaxed standing posture supporting the gravitational line with the normal knee locked position, which muscles are used for balance?
   a. Psoas
   b. Gastrocnemius
   c. Hamstrings
   d. Quadriceps

_____ 12. A massage professional is complaining of pain in the wrist in an area near the elbow. Which of the following is an appropriate corrective action?
   a. Maintain the hands in a clenched fist to promote stability.
   b. Increase the movement of the stoke at the shoulder joint.
   c. Relax the hand and fingers during massage.
   d. Shift the compressive force to the fingers and thumb.

_____ 13. Observation of a fellow massage practitioner reveals that he or she has the shoulder girdle in alignment with the pelvic girdle, the pressure-bearing arm opposite the weight-bearing leg, fingers relaxed, head up, back straight, elbows bent, and stance asymmetrical. Which of these areas need correction?
   a. Elbows
   b. Stance
   c. Back position
   d. Shoulder position

_____ 14. When stretching the legs of a client, the massage practitioner should perform which one of the following?
   a. Fix the feet and pull with the shoulders.
   b. Move to a symmetrical stance and lean back.
   c. Lean back keeping the back straight.
   d. Bend the knees and push back.

Preparation for Massage: Equipment, Supplies, Professional Environment, Positioning, and Draping

▼ INSTRUCTOR OBJECTIVES

1. List equipment, supplies, and setup of location needed to begin a massage practice.
2. Discuss pros and cons of the various types of equipment necessary for developing a massage setting in different types of environments.
3. Demonstrate methods for the care and protection of the student's hands and his or her general health.
4. Present information to assist the student in making informed decisions about purchasing a massage table, chair, mat, body supports, draping materials, and lubricants. Present pros and cons relative to these decisions.
5. Demonstrate effective use of massage equipment.
6. Discuss methods to present massage procedures to clients.
7. Demonstrate how to interview a new client to better understand the client's expectations of massage in general and the outcome for a massage session in particular.

8. Demonstrate how to elicit feedback from the client.
9. Demonstrate how to provide appropriate feedback to the client.
10. Discuss differences in expectations and interpretation of touch based on gender.
11. Provide the structure for an orientation process for a new client.
12. Present methods appropriate for focusing and centering.
13. Demonstrate effective draping and positioning of the client.
14. Position, drape, and perform a massage session in four basic positions.
15. Demonstrate how to drape effectively with two basic styles.

CHAPTER SUMMARY

This chapter helps the therapeutic massage professional develop the important premassage procedures that support the therapeutic relationship and professional environment first discussed in Chapter 2. This chapter focuses on certain preparations that must be done before the massage begins, including room setup, types of supplies and equipment, centering to help focus on the client and the session, client positioning, draping procedures, history taking, assessment procedures, and feedback.

CHAPTER HIGHLIGHTS AND POINTS FOR DISCUSSION

The most important pieces of massage equipment are the massage professional's hands and body.

Discuss the self-care recommendations in this chapter and review the importance of body mechanics discussed in Chapter 7.

A massage table must be sturdy and properly assembled to ensure that it will not collapse when a client is laying on it. Two basic types of table are the portable table, which folds into a smaller unit and is easily moved from place to place, and the stationary table, which remains in one location.

Special massage chairs are available for seated massage.

Some methods of massage are performed on a mat on the floor.

Body supports are used to bolster the body during the massage and to provide contour to the flat working surface.

Discuss the pros and cons of the various forms of equipment.

Demonstrate the various forms of equipment.

The purpose of using an opaque draping material is to provide the client with privacy and warmth. The most common coverings are standard bed linens because they are large enough to cover the entire body and are easily used for most draping procedures.

Large towels may be used for draping because they are both warm and opaque. An alternative is to use sheets and towels in combination with a bath-size towel as a chest covering. Disposable linen is also available.

Discuss the pros and cons of the various forms of draping material. Demonstrate the use of various forms of draping material.

Lubricants reduce friction on the skin during gliding-type massage strokes. Medicinal and cosmetic use of lubricants is beyond the scope of practice for therapeutic massage. Avoid using scented lubricant products. Lubricants are classified as oils, creams, or powders.

Very little lubricant needs to be used when giving a massage. More lubricant is required to work over body hair. In some cases, powder may be a better choice. Occasionally, the use of all lubricants is contraindicated, thus the massage professional must be able to do massage without using lubricants.

Do not pour lubricant directly on the client. The lubricant is first warmed in the palms of the practitioner's hands by rubbing them together. Apply to one area at a time as opposed to the entire body. Avoid using lubricant on the face and hair because it disturbs makeup and hairstyles.

Discuss the pros and cons of the various forms of lubricants. Demonstrate the use of various forms of lubricants.

In addition to a massage table, draping material, supports, and lubricants, disposable tissues, a clock, and music are desirable to have available.

Clients will return for a massage because they appreciate the quality of the service and a professional personality and environment.

General conditions for massage areas that need to be considered are the room temperature, fresh air supply, privacy, and accessibility.

Many clients are also environmentally sensitive and react to scents, incense, and flowers. The best recommendation is to avoid using these items because the fragrance lingers and can cause problems for a client.

Discuss the importance of the massage environment in terms of the previous criteria.

The massage professional must attend to personal hygiene and prevent body odors because people are sensitive to these smells. Avoid heavy use of aftershave, perfume, scented cosmetic products, or hair spray. Clients will not usually comment on offensive breath or body odors; they just may not return for further sessions.

Hands should be heated with warm water, on a hot water bottle, or by rubbing them together before touching the client.

Discuss personal hygiene and using scented products and any other issues involving smell and temperature.

Various locations are used to provide massage. These areas include a private office, public setting, on-site residence, and outdoors. A massage area separate from the business area in the massage setting should be designated.

Discuss the pros and cons of each massage setting.

The massage practitioner should carefully explain the limitations of massage to the client, put into perspective the expectations, and help define the outcome for the massage. These aspects should be covered in the beginning as part of informed consent procedures before the massage begins. This information is first presented in Chapter 2.

If the client has never had a massage, expectations will be determined by what has been heard, read, or observed. The massage practitioner should explain the different approaches that are used so the client is not on the table wondering why this massage is so different from what was expected.

The outcome for massage is what the client can anticipate in response to the benefits in the proposed massage plan.

Explain massage procedures in detail in a manner that the client can understand.

Discuss and demonstrate the way to explain limits, expectations, and outcomes to a client.

Feedback is a noninvasive and ongoing exchange of information between the client and the professional. Feedback is not social conversation; it is common for a client to talk during the massage and appropriate for a massage professional to listen to the client while remaining focused on the massage. *Engaging in social conversation with clients, particularly regarding the client's personal life, is inappropriate for the professional.*

Discuss the components of feedback and what constitutes appropriate and inappropriate professional conversation.

Gender influences the professional interaction. Male and female professionals may experience some difference in the client's expectation and interpretation of touch.

Discuss potential gender issues. Refer to Chapter 1 for a review of interpretation of touch.

After the initial intake process, the new client is ready to enter the massage room. The new client should be given an orientation of the area.

Do not assume that a client remembers the instructions or has knowledge of what to do or what is expected. Explain all steps in detail.

Discuss and demonstrate an orientation process.

While waiting for the client to prepare for the massage, the practitioner should also prepare. The goal is to be present in the moment for the client and not focused on lists of things that need to be done. If a routine sequence for focusing is developed, the practitioner will become calm and centered much faster.

Discuss and demonstrate various centering procedures. The basic positions for massage are supine (face up), prone (face down), side lying, and seated.

Discuss the pros and cons of each position, especially in relation to body mechanics and client comfort. Demonstrate each method of positioning with bolstering.

Draping has two purposes:
1. Maintaining client privacy and sense of security
2. Warmth

The client can be draped in many ways. The main principles during draping include the following:

- All draping material must be freshly laundered using a bleach or other approved solution.
- Only the area being massaged is undraped.
- The genital area is never undraped. The breast area of women is not undraped during routine wellness massage. Specific medical massage under the supervision of a licensed medical professional may require special draping procedures for the female breast area. Males and females should be draped the same to avoid allegations of discrimination.
- Draping methods should cover the client in all positions, including the seated position.

Discuss and demonstrate the various draping methods. Use the illustrations and available video from Mosby (*Mosby's Fundamentals of Therapeutic Massage* videotape series, video 1, Massage Overview and Draping Procedures) to support the instruction.

After the massage is complete, do not linger in conversation. The attitude in the business area is one of polite and courteous completion. After the client leaves, the practitioner must update all records, prepare the room for the next client, and attend to personal hygiene and self-care.

Discuss postmassage procedures, including closure with the client at the end of the massage.

Review record keeping from Chapter 3.

MULTIPLE-CHOICE TEST BANK

_____ 1. A massage mat:
   a. Is usually more expensive than a table
   b. Is often heavier than a table
   c. Is portable
   d. Should not be used when working with children

_____ 2. When choosing a portable table, a necessary feature is:
   a. A width of less than 22 inches
   b. Sturdy construction
   c. An electric height adjustment
   d. A solid top with no hinge

_____ 3. Lubricants:
a. Include minerals and petroleum
b. Do not cause respiratory problems
c. Should be heated then poured onto the client
d. **Reduce friction on the skin**

_____ 4. The massage site:
a. **Should be separate from the business area**
b. Must have a floor plan
c. Includes a separate room for the business area
d. Is located in either an office or fitness establishment

_____ 5. A way of distracting a client from surrounding noise is by using:
a. A loud clock
b. Candles or incense
c. **Appropriate music**
d. Conversation during the session

_____ 6. The outcome for massage:
a. Is the same as the client's expectations
b. Is to be solely determined by the client
c. Depends mainly on the length of the session
d. **Is what the client can anticipate in response to the proposed plan**

_____ 7. When positioning and draping the client:
a. **Only the area being massaged is undraped.**
b. All draping material is to be discarded after the session.
c. Use sheets instead of towels.
d. Avoid moving the client because this disturbs the outcome.

_____ 8. If a client is left alone at the end of the session, remind him or her to:
a. Roll onto the stomach.
b. **Sit for a minute before getting up.**
c. Push the arms to a seated position.
d. Return the seat to an upright position.

_____ 9. Contoured draping:
a. **Can be done with the client's assistance**
b. Requires the use of fitted sheets
c. Cannot be done with towels
d. Is best done with a client in a swimsuit or shorts

_____ 10. Feedback is:
a. Social conversation used to distract a client from surrounding noise
b. Gender-specific in terms of the types of questions to be asked and information dispensed
c. **A noninvasive and ongoing exchange of information between the client and the professional**
d. Limited in terms of the amount of talking by the client and primarily the responsibility of the professional

_____ 11. To prevent allergic reaction all lubricants should be:
a. Oil based
b. Water based
c. Dispensed in sanitary fashion
d. **Scent free**

_____ 12. In which situation would you stay in the massage room and assist a client on and off the massage table?
a. First trimester pregnancy
b. 65-year-old man with diabetes
c. **Older woman with high blood pressure**
d. Adolescent with a wrist cast

_____ 13. A client regularly lingers after the massage session to talk. The massage professional becomes behind in the schedule as a result. What is the most likely cause of this problem?
a. **Policies regarding leaving promptly after the massage were not addressed and reinforced.**
b. The client requires a longer appointment.
c. The client needs more frequent appointments.
d. The massage professional is displaying transference.

Massage Manipulations and Techniques

GENERAL MASSAGE SUGGESTIONS
   Body hair
   Skin problems
   Avoidance of tickling
   Considerations and suggestions for massage
     applications by body region
     Considerations and suggestions for head and face
      massage
     Considerations and suggestions for neck massage
     Considerations and suggestions for shoulder massage
     Considerations and suggestions for arm massage
     Considerations and suggestions for hand/wrist massage
     Considerations and suggestions for chest massage
     Considerations and suggestions for abdominal massage
     Considerations and suggestions for back massage
     Considerations and suggestions for gluteal/hip massage
     Considerations and suggestions for leg massage
     Considerations and suggestions for foot/ankle massage
SUMMARY

▼INSTRUCTOROBJECTIVES

1. Present the basic theories for the physiologic effects of massage methods and techniques.
2. Categorize the effects of massage methods and techniques into *stimulating* or *inhibiting* physiologic responses.
3. Evaluate massage manipulations based on seven criteria.
4. Classify massage manipulations and techniques into three categories based on reflexive, mechanical, and chemical effects.
5. Discuss and demonstrate how to establish and adjust the physical contact with the client effectively.
6. Demonstrate how to organize massage methods and techniques into basic flow patterns.
7. Demonstrate how to use a specific massage pattern on the abdomen.
8. Demonstrate how to perform eight basic massage manipulations.
9. Demonstrate how to combine the eight massage manipulations into a basic full-body massage.
10. Demonstrate how to use movement in a purposeful way to create a specific physiologic response.
11. Explain the proprioceptive mechanisms and their importance in the physiologic effects of massage techniques. For an additional scientific explanation, refer to *Mosby's Essential Sciences for Therapeutic Massage: Anatomy, Physiology, Biomechanics, and Pathology,* second edition, Chapter 5 and Chapter 8.
12. Demonstrate how to move the synovial joints through the client's physiologic range of motion using both active and passive joint movement.
13. Demonstrate how to incorporate muscle energy techniques to enhance lengthening and stretching proce-

dures. Review *Mosby's Essential Sciences* activities in Chapter 10 regarding muscle energy techniques.
14. Discuss the pros and cons of each massage method and technique.
15. Demonstrate how to perform a full-body massage using the methods and techniques presented.
16. Explain the importance of massage variation using the clinical reasoning process. See *Mosby's Essential Sciences,* Chapter 10. Use the *Fundamentals* textbook Chapter 15 as a guide when assessing and developing treatment plans.

CHAPTER SUMMARY

This core technical chapter includes definitions, descriptions, and directions for the applications and uses of the most common massage methods and techniques. The student must understand both why and where massage methods and techniques are used, as well as how to organize a process that uses the various therapeutic approaches efficiently. The chapter examines each of the individual massage manipulations and techniques.

CHAPTER HIGHLIGHTS AND POINTS FOR DISCUSSION

All massage methods use some form of external sensory stimulation or application of force that can stimulate or inhibit body processes, depending on their use. Some methods work better with mechanical effects, others with reflexive effects, and still others are better at initiating chemical responses. In general, fast, specific applications of a method tend to stimulate, whereas slow general applications tend to inhibit.

Generalizing the mechanical, reflexive, or chemical effect of massage manipulations and techniques is not easy. Frequently, the combination of the effects of massage, coupled with the client's psychologic state and receptivity to the massage, causes the response.

Discuss the importance of understanding the physiology of massage manipulations in terms of making decisions with regard to which methods to choose to achieve a specific outcome.

The following components for the quality of touch are considered in the textbook. Individual massage methods vary in relation to the depth of pressure, drag, direction, speed, rhythm, frequency, and duration.

Discuss how the infinite variations in application of massage can be derived from using basic methods by adjusting the components of quality of touch.

The massage practitioner must make contact with the client's body in a secure and confident way. Once physical contact has been made with the client and the massage has begun, the intention of the contact should not be broken, meaning that the massage practitioner must remain focused on the client for the entire session. Maintaining contact does not mean that the practitioner never removes his or her hands from the client.

Discuss what is meant by the intention of contact.

The four patterns that cover the client's position are prone, supine, lying on his or her side, and seated. The sequence used on the abdomen always remains the same.

Review the pros and cons of each position in terms of body mechanics, draping, and client comfort.

Albert Baumgartner, in his 1947 book *Massage in Athletics,* quotes Plato as saying "Massage must be simple." Discuss this quote.

All massage can be categorized as the application of a stimulus (reflex) that affects the neuroendocrine response or the application of a force that mechanically affects tissue. Forces applied are tension, compression, bend, shear, and torsion.

Massage Manipulations

Discuss and demonstrate each of the following massage manipulations. Encourage variations in applications. Use the illustrations in this chapter to support instruction.

Resting Position

The act of placing your hands on another person seems so simple, but this initial contact must be made with respect and a client-centered focus.

Gliding Strokes or Effleurage

The full spectrum of effleurage is determined by pressure, drag, speed, direction, and rhythm, making this manipulation one of the most versatile.

Kneading or Pétrissage

Pétrissage requires that the soft tissue be lifted, rolled, and squeezed by the massage technician.

Skin Rolling

A variation of this lifting manipulation is skin rolling. In this technique, only the skin is lifted from the underlying muscle layer.

Compression

The focus of compression is a vertical pressing down. Because compression uses a lift-press method, it is particularly suited for use when a lubricant is undesirable.

Vibration

The focus of vibration is down and back and forth in a fast, oscillating manner.

Shaking

Shaking begins with a lift-and-pull component. Either a muscle group or limb is grasped, lifted, and shaken. To begin to understand shaking, think of how a dog shakes when it is wet, shaking out a rug or blanket, what a dog or cat does when tugging on a toy, or the swish of a horse's tail.

Rocking

Rocking is a soothing and rhythmic method that has been used since the beginning of time to calm people.

Rocking is rhythmic and should be applied with a deliberate full-body movement. Rocking involves the up-and-down and side-to-side movement of shaking, but no flick or throw-off snap occurs at the end of the movement.

Percussion or Tapotement

Tapotement techniques require that the hands or parts of the hand administer springy blows to the body at a fast rate. The blows are directed downward to create a rhythmic compression of the tissue:

1. Hacking
2. Cupping
3. Fist beating
4. Beating over palm
5. Slapping
6. Finger tapping

Friction

One method of *friction* consists of small deep movements performed on a local area. Friction creates therapeutic inflammation. A modified application of friction, used to keep high-concentration areas of connective tissue soft and pliable, is appropriate for the beginner. The modified application is essentially the same as deep transverse friction in that the focus is transverse to the muscle fiber direction and moves the tissue beneath the skin, but the duration and specificity are reduced.

Massage Techniques

Discuss and demonstrate each of the following massage techniques. Encourage variations in applications, but be attentive to anatomic influences to positioning and the importance of the specific isolation of muscles and proper stabilization. Use the illustrations in this chapter to support instruction.

The Textbook

The techniques of passive and active joint movement (muscle energy) presented in the textbook work with the neuromuscular reflex system to relax and *lengthen* muscles. In contrast, *stretching* has both a reflexive and mechanical aspect. The reflexive component of stretching is an initial neuromuscular lengthening phase used to prepare the area for the more mechanical stretching effect of elongating connective tissue. Stretching is discussed more completely in the text.

Joint Movement

Joints have various degrees of range of motion. Anatomic, physiologic, and pathologic barriers to motion exist. Discuss and demonstrate each of these motion barriers.

Joint End-Feel

When a normal joint is taken to its physiologic limit, a bit more movement—a sort of springiness in the joint—is usually possible. This springiness is called a *soft end-feel*.

When abnormal restriction is present, the limit does not have any spring, as found at a physiologic barrier. However, similar to a jammed door or drawer, the joint is fixed at the barrier, and any attempt to take it farther is uncomfortable and distinctly "binding" or jamming, rather than springy. This binding is called a *hard end-feel*.

Discuss and demonstrate soft and hard end-feel. (Elbow extension is a good example of hard end-feel.) Discuss the importance of anatomic and physiologic instruction to be able to perform these methods.

Joint movement is effective because it provides a means of controlled stimulation to the joint mechanoreceptors. Movement initiates muscle tension readjustment through the reflex center of the spinal cord and lower brain centers. Joint movement also encourages lubrication of the joint and adds an important addition to the lymphatic and venous circulation enhancement systems. Remember that each person is unique, and many factors influence available range of motion.

Types of Joint Movement Methods

The two types of joint movement are active and passive. Working within the physiologic ranges of motion for each particular client is within the scope of practice of the massage professional. Specific corrective procedures for pathologic range of motion are best applied in a supervised heath care setting.

Joint Movement's Relationship to Lengthening and Stretching Methods

Joint movement facilitates the application of muscle energy techniques to lengthen muscles, as well as stretching methods for elongating connective tissues.

Hand placement with joint movement is very important. Make sure that the area is not squeezed, pinched, or restricted in its movement pattern. One hand should be placed close to the joint to be moved so that it acts as a stabilizer and allows for evaluation. The practitioner's other hand is placed at the distal end of the bone and is the hand that actually provides the movement. Proper use of body mechanics is essential when using joint movement. Stabilization must occur, otherwise the therapeutic benefit of joint movement methods is diminished.

In *active range of motion,* the client moves the jointed area without any type of interaction by the massage practitioner. In active-assistive range of motion, the client moves the joint through the range of motion, and the therapist helps or assists the movement.

In *active-resisted range of motion,* the massage therapist resists the movement while the client initiates movement.

To perform *passive range of motion,* instruct the client to relax the area by letting it lie heavily in your hands. Slowly and rhythmically move the joint through a comfortable range of motion for the jointed area. Repeat the action three or more times, increasing the limits of the range of motion as the muscles relax.

Muscle energy methods emerged from the osteopathic profession. *Muscle energy techniques* involve a voluntary contraction of the client's muscle in a specific and controlled direction, at varying levels of intensity, against a specific counterforce that the massage practitioner applies. Muscle energy procedures have a variety of applications and are considered active techniques in which the client contributes the corrective force. Muscle energy techniques are focused on specific muscles or muscle groups. The massage practitioner must position muscles so that the origin and insertion are either close together or in a lengthening phase with the origin and insertion separated.

NOTE: **Review the muscle testing activities regarding positioning for muscle energy techniques in** *Mosby's Essential Sciences,* **Chapter 10.**

Discuss the importance of anatomy and physiology instruction to performing these methods.

The massage therapist uses three different types of muscle contractions to activate muscle energy techniques: *sometric contraction, isotonic contraction, and multiple isotonic contractions.*

Two neurophysiologic principles explain the effect of the techniques as a result of physiologic laws being applied, not from mechanical force, as in stretching. These principles are postisometric relaxation (PIR) and reciprocal inhibition (RI). PIR (tense and relax) and RI can be combined to enhance the lengthening effects.

Pulsed muscle energy procedures involve engaging the comfort barrier and using small, resisted contractions (usually 20 in 10 seconds), which introduces mechanical pumping, as well as PIR or RI, depending on the muscles used.

Direct Applications

The principles of muscle energy techniques can be used by direct manipulation of the spindle cells or Golgi tendons. Pushing muscle fibers together in the direction of the fibers in the belly of a muscle weakens the muscle by working with the spindle cells.

Separating the muscle fibers in the belly of the muscle in the direction of the fibers strengthens the muscle. The same responses can be obtained by using the Golgi tendon organs, except that the manipulation of the proprioception signal cells is reversed. Manipulation of the Golgi tendon organs is at the ends of the muscle where it joins the tendons. To weaken the muscle, pull apart on the tendon attachments of the target muscle. To strengthen the muscle, push the tendon attachments together. The pressure levels used to elicit the response need to be sufficient to contract the muscle fibers. Too light of a pressure will not access the proprioceptors. Excessive pressure will negate the response by activating protective reflexes. *Applying moderate pressure where the muscle itself can be palpated is most effective.*

Positional Release

Strain-counter strain was formalized by Dr. Lawrence Jones and involves using tender points to guide the positioning of the body into a space where the muscle tension can release on its own.

The positioning used during positional release is a full-body process. Remember, an injury or loss of balance is a full-body experience. Thus areas distant to the tender point must be considered during the positioning process. The position of the feet may have an effect on a tender point in the neck.

Muscle energy methods can be used together or in sequence to enhance their effects.

Stretching is a mechanical method of pulling connective tissue to reduce tensile stress and elongate areas of shortened connective tissue. Stretching affects the fiber component of connective tissue by elongating the fibers past the normal give of the fiber to enter the plastic range past the existing bind.

Stretching and lengthening are different. Before any stretching is attempted, lengthening must be done or the muscles of the area may develop protective spasms, because stretching often moves into pathologic barriers formed by connective tissue changes. The connective tissue component cannot be accessed until the muscle is lengthened. Without stretching, any neuromuscular lengthening may be restricted by shortened connective tissue. Although lengthening without stretching is possible and often desirable, lengthening before stretching is always necessary. During stretching, the two methods work in conjunction with each other. Muscle energy techniques are used to prepare muscles to stretch by activating lengthening responses.

Longitudinal stretching pulls connective tissue in the direction of the fiber configuration. *Cross-directional stretching* pulls the connective tissue against the fiber direction.

Massage Variations

A massage may be given in many ways, and the decisions made each time a massage is given develop from an understanding of the principles and practice of therapeutic massage. Each massage is different because the client is different each time, even if the client has been seen for many massage sessions.

The basic full-body massage is a common approach in massage. The full-body general massage stimulates all of the sensory nerve receptors, contacts all of the layers and types of tissues, and moves all of the major joints of the body. The session lasts approximately 1 hour. A protocol is presented in the text and on Box 9-2 on page 36, but should not be enforced as the only way to perform massage.

Discuss and demonstrate each method and technique in terms of pros and cons of application. For example, gliding methods are effective for moving body fluids but require using a lubricant. Compression does not require a lubricant but may feel more choppy to the client. Kneading is effective in softening superficial fascial but is energy-expending and hard on the hands of the practitioner. Percussion is most effective at the musculotendinous junction if the goal is to affect proprioceptive receptors. Percussion is less effective if attempting to stimulate a parasympathetic response. Each instructor has worked with the methods sufficiently to be able to help the students logically analyze when a particular approach is effective.

Discuss the importance of the clinical reasoning process in relation to decision making regarding choosing among the various methods and techniques when designing a particular massage session.

MULTIPLE-CHOICE TEST BANK

_____ 1. Muscle-energy techniques:
  a. Are considered passive techniques
  b. Involve a voluntary contraction of a muscle against a counterforce
  c. Are applied in an abrupt manner to release tight muscles
  d. Do not require muscles to be in a specific position

_____ 2. Friction:
   a. Should be done with adequate lubricant
   b. Should be done with acute injuries or fresh scars
   c. Increases pain through counterirritation
   d. Loosens or breaks up adhesions by creating controlled inflammation

_____ 3. Joint movement:
   a. Should be performed smoothly and evenly
   b. Should be performed only while the client is in the supine position
   c. Is contraindicated when the client is an older adult
   d. Will result in temporary pain

_____ 4. Mechanical methods:
   a. Add sensory stimulation to cause the nervous system to respond
   b. Have a direct effect on the tissues
   c. Account for a majority of benefit derived from massage
   d. Are limited to methods that use electrical devices

_____ 5. Gliding strokes:
   a. Can be superficial or deep
   b. Is the least versatile of the strokes and the most limiting
   c. Is applied vertically in relation to the tissues
   d. Is performed with the fingertips to be most effective

_____ 6. Rocking:
   a. Is a form of pétrissage
   b. Should be repeated only two or three times during the massage
   c. Should not be used on the whole body
   d. Is reflexive and chemical in its effects

_____ 7. Skin rolling:
   a. Is as valuable as a caliper test for determining body fat percentage
   b. Is applied rapidly for the best results
   c. Is a valuable connective-tissue technique
   d. Is most often used on the tissues of the face

_____ 8. Stretching:
   a. Is a mechanical force applied to increase pliability in connective tissues
   b. Is the same as lengthening
   c. Is done to firm and tighten muscles
   d. Does not address connective tissue areas

_____ 9. Postisometric relaxation:
   a. Is the refractory period of a muscle
   b. Follows an isometric contraction
   c. Lasts up to 30 minutes
   d. Works against gravity

_____ 10. Performing a massage routine:
   a. Is a good approach because all clients received the same care
   b. Does not teach the value of sequence and general flow
   c. Seldom meets the outcomes of most clients
   d. Is a good learning method but must be modified to fit the client

_____ 11. When the outcome for the massage is to produce parasympathetic dominance, which combination of methods would be the best choice?
   a. Gliding, rocking, and passive joint movement
   b. Compression, shaking, and friction
   c. Active joint movement, reciprocal inhibition, and rocking
   d. Tapotement, compression, and vibration

_____ 12. A client complains of restricted range of motion in the shoulder. The primary outcome for the massage is to increase shoulder mobility. Which method would be the best choice?
   a. Friction
   b. Muscle energy
   c. Hydrotherapy
   d. Resting stroke

_____ 13. A client complains of a stiff and stuck feeling in the lumbar area. Assessment indicates that the fascia in that area is thick and adhered to the underlying tissue. Which method would best restore pliability to this tissue?
   a. Skin rolling
   b. Shaking
   c. Friction
   d. Vibration

_____ 14. Which of the following body areas is often massaged longer than what is effective?
   a. Hands
   b. Abdomen
   c. Legs
   d. Back

_____ 15. A client arrives late for a massage appointment. The remaining time is 30 minutes. The goal for the session is general relaxation. Which combination is the best choice to achieve desired outcomes in the allotted time?
   a. Back, gluteals, and hips
   b. Face, hands, and feet
   c. Hands, arms, and back
   d. Face, neck, and shoulders

_____ 16. Why is care taken when massaging the face?
   a. Proximity to mucous membranes and transmission of pathogens
   b. The skin of the face is thin.
   c. Facial muscles are weak.
   d. Compression damages underlying cranial sutures.

Assessment Procedures for Developing a Care Plan

Muscular imbalance, muscle testing, and functional assessment
Range of motion
Compensation patterns
Dysfunction as a solution
CLINICAL REASONING AND PROBLEM SOLVING TO CREATE MASSAGE CARE/TREATMENT PLANS
Care or treatment plan
Reassessment
SUMMARY

▼INSTRUCTOROBJECTIVES

1. Demonstrate how to conduct an effective client interview.
2. Present and demonstrate how to complete a basic physical assessment, gait assessment, 14-level palpation assessment, and muscle testing assessment. Also review Chapter 8 for palpation of joints and Chapter 10 for gait cycle in *Mosby's Essential Sciences for Therapeutic Massage: Anatomy, Physiology, Biomechanics, and Pathology,* second edition.
3. Discuss how to interpret assessment information and develop a care or treatment plan.
4. Discuss how to interpret assessment information for the purpose of designing a basic full-body massage session focused on the specific outcome desired by the client.

NOTE: **Section Four opener in *Mosby's Essential Sciences* has a clinical reasoning activity example that should also be reviewed to assist the student in recognizing different types of massage approaches.**

5. Present criteria for referring clients for care when the assessment information indicates the need for specific diagnosis and treatment.
6. Demonstrate and reinforce how to use the clinical reasoning model as a decision-making tool in developing massage care or treatment plans.
7. Demonstrate and reinforce how to use the clinical reasoning model to choose specific massage approaches to use as intervention methods during the massage session.

CHAPTER SUMMARY

This chapter corresponds with Chapter 10 in *Mosby's Essential Sciences* and teaches the student to perform an assessment and develop an individual care plan.

Being able to reason clinically supports the effectiveness of all massage interaction, whether for relaxation and pleasure or for managing complex conditions in con-

junction with medical interventions. Because most physiologic changes and benefits of massage occur from the most basic of technical skills, the expertise comes from the decisions made in applying these skills. The ability to make these decisions depends on the ability to gather client historical data, perform physical assessment and analysis, and interpret the information. This chapter consolidates the information gathering, decision making, and plan development first presented in previous chapters. At this point, the student is advanced enough to make practical use of the skills developed in these chapters. This chapter can be considered the integration chapter in which professional skill comes together with technical skills in the therapeutic relationship. This chapter demonstrates competency-based learning (see Rubric in the Appendix).

CHAPTER HIGHLIGHTS AND POINTS FOR DISCUSSION

Assessment is the collection and interpretation of information that the client provides, the client's consent advocates (parent or guardian), and the referring medical professionals, as well as from information that the massage practitioner gathers.

In more clinical health care settings, assessment by the massage professional is considered in the total treatment plan developed in cooperation with the client's multidisciplinary health care team. Therefore the massage practitioner needs to understand and practice standard assessment and charting procedures.

Discuss the components of standardized assessment and charting procedures. Refer to Chapter 3.

Assessment does not change a condition but instead seeks to understand it. Interventions cause change. The student must learn to separate assessment information obtained before, during, and after the massage from intervention methods to be able to understand and analyze the results that the massage session achieves. In terms of communication, assessment is listening, or receiving information, and intervention is talking, or delivering information.

Discuss the difference between assessment and intervention. Review communication skills in Chapter 2 as a metaphor, depicting assessment as listening and intervention as talking. Discuss how the same massage methods can accomplish the two approaches; for example, effleurage or gliding strokes can both assess tissue texture and be used to alter tissue texture.

The client is the most important resource during the assessment process. The skills required of the massage professional during this process are the ability to establish rapport, keen observation, successful interviewing methods, and active listening.

Communication skills are actively used during interviewing procedures and throughout client-practitioner interactions. Review communication skills in Chapter 2.

Discuss and review the forms in Chapter 3 when teaching assessment procedures. This chapter should provide a more integrated understanding of using these forms.

Assessment for a basic therapeutic massage with treatment plan development and agreed-on outcomes for the massage includes a general evaluation of the client's posture and gait (walking pattern). During physical assessment, the main considerations are body balance, efficient function, and basic symmetry.

Three major factors influence posture include heredity, disease, and habit.

The standing posture requires various segments of the body to cooperate mechanically as a whole.

Understanding the basic body movements of walking will help the massage practitioner recognize dysfunctional and inefficient gait patterns. Any disruption of the gait demands that the body compensate by shifting movement patterns and posture. Because of this characteristic, all dysfunctional patterns are whole-body phenomena. Working only on the area of symptoms is ineffective and offers limited relief.

When dealing with palpation assessment, the main considerations for basic massage are the ability to differentiate among different types of tissue and the ability to distinguish differences of tissue texture within the same tissue types. Palpation includes assessment for hot and cold and observation of skin color and general skin condition. Palpation also assesses various body rhythms, including breathing patterns and pulses. The tissues with which the massage therapist should be concerned and should be able to distinguish are skin, superficial fascia, fascial sheaths, tendons, ligaments, blood vessels, muscles, and bone. Chapter 9 in *Mosby's Essential Sciences* provides additional information on palpating muscles.

Discuss and demonstrate assessment of the previously mentioned tissues.

Muscle testing procedures are used for different purposes. *Strength testing* seeks to discover whether the muscle being tested is responding with sufficient strength to perform the required body functions. *Neurologic muscle testing* seeks to discover whether the neurologic interaction of the muscles is working smoothly.

Discuss the different types of information obtained by these two muscle tests. Discuss muscle firing sequence and gait assessment and the relevance to massage.

The two basic types of muscles are those that support the body in gravity and those that move it against gravity. Muscles that support the body in gravity are called *postural muscles,* and those that move the body against gravity are called *phasic muscles.*

Discuss the different muscle types in relation to application of assessment and intervention methods. For example, postural muscles take longer than phasic muscles to fatigue with direct pressure methods when dealing with trigger points.

Once the information has been gathered, an interpretation and analysis process is used to develop the best massage plan for the individual client. This process requires clinical reasoning and problem-solving skills.

Reinforce, discuss, and demonstrate the analysis process.

The importance of compensation needs to be considered. Many instances of *resourceful compensation* occur in which the body has made adjustments to manage a permanent or chronic dysfunction. The concept of dysfunction as a solution is similar to the patterns of resourceful compensation. If all the information gathered during assessment can be viewed as *an attempt at a solution,* a broader perspective is created in the decision making required for effective massage care plans.

Discuss various forms of compensation in relation to treatment plan development, determination of outcome goals, and decisions about the types of massage approaches used.

Effective work with clients becomes an ongoing learning process of assessment, determining intervention procedures, analyzing effectiveness by a postassessment process, and recognizing progress made from session to session. Even in the most basic of sessions with clients, the goals of pleasure and relaxation still require decisions to be made regarding how best to encourage the body to respond to meet the particular client's goals.

Discuss the importance of individualizing each massage session and the role of clinical reasoning for decision making in this process. Review the concepts of therapeutic change, condition management, and palliative care.

MULTIPLE-CHOICE TEST BANK

_____ 1. Information gathered during assessment:
   a. Helps develop the massage plan
   b. Helps the massage professional diagnose the condition
   c. Helps determine outcomes but not massage application
   d. Is not often shared with the client

_____ 2. Information the client provides is considered:
   a. Of little value in the massage
   b. Objective assessment
   c. The application of information
   d. Subjective assessment

3. For basic massage, the physical assessment is often limited to:
   a. Things heard and seen but not recorded
   b. Having the client demonstrate restricted or painful movements
   c. Checking a client's size and balance
   d. Determining connective tissue dysfunction

4. Many physical compensation patterns are in response to:
   a. New shoes or clothing
   b. Telephone habits
   c. The body's attempt to adapt
   d. Supportive furniture

5. When assessing posture in the standing client:
   a. The symmetrical stance must be used.
   b. The feet must be together.
   c. The asymmetrical stance must be used.
   d. The therapist squats to view the legs and knees.

6. A good indicator of a dysfunctional area during walking:
   a. Is the areas that move in a figure-8 pattern
   b. Is heel strike
   c. Reminds the therapist to work on the area of symptoms
   d. Is an area of the body that either does not move or moves too much

7. Postural muscles:
   a. Move the body when upright
   b. Rarely contain trigger points
   c. Primarily produce movement
   d. Hold contractions for long periods

8. When a client is functioning under sympathetic autonomic nervous system activation, the massage should:
   a. Initially begin with relaxation methods
   b. Start with stimulating techniques
   c. Use slow rocking to begin
   d. Not discharge energy

9. With posture assessment:
   a. Remember not to exaggerate the pattern.
   b. Asymmetry is caused by gravity.
   c. The focus is symmetry.
   d. Push or pull the client.

10. Skeletal muscle tissue that is firm and pliable:
    a. Is usually healthy and normal
    b. Indicates connective tissue dysfunction
    c. Shows muscle atrophy
    d. Shows muscle hypertrophy

11. Which of the following is part of a normal gait pattern?
    a. The arms swing freely opposite the leg swing.
    b. The knee is maintained in the "screw home" mechanism.
    c. The toes contact the floor first and then roll to the heel.
    d. During push off, the foot is dorsiflexed.

12. When observing for symmetry, which of the following is correct?
    a. The shoulders should evenly roll forward, leveling the clavicles.
    b. The circumference of the muscle mass in the legs should be similar.
    c. The ribs should be fixed more on the left and springy on the right.
    d. The patella should be pointed more medially.

13. A vacationing client will only have one massage from the massage practitioner. Which is the appropriate assessment process?
    a. Subjective history taking for possible referral combined with a physical assessment for symmetry and gait assessment for optimal movement patterns
    b. Palpation assessment of soft tissues to identify treatment areas
    c. Subjective and objective assessment for contraindications
    d. Interviewing for client's quantitative goals

14. A client is experiencing spasms in the left thigh flexor muscles. An attempt to muscle test the area might result in a cramp. The massage professional remembers that activating gait reflexes can either facilitate or inhibit muscle contraction of other muscles in the pattern. Which group of muscles would the massage professional have the client contract to inhibit the left thigh flexors?
    a. The left arm flexors
    b. The right arm flexors
    c. The left arm extensors
    d. The right thigh extensors

_____ 15. A client is referred for massage by her physician for circulation enhancement to the limbs. The client complains of experiencing cold hands and feet. Assessment indicates decreased pliability of the tissues around the elbows and knees. Work-related activities require repetitive movement in these areas. The massage professional considers three main approaches for the physician to consider:
1. General massage and rest
2. General massage with connective tissue stretching in the restricted areas
3. Compression focused specifically to the arteries to encourage circulation

Considering all three options, the massage professional eliminates option 1 as too time consuming. Option 2 seems viable, but the client does not respond well to methods that may be painful. Option 3 seems limited in the approach to the massage profession. The decision is to begin with option 3 and expand to connective tissue methods when the client is able to tolerate them. Which part of this process best reflects brainstorming possibilities?
a. Data collection
b. Eliminations of options based on pros and cons
c. **Generating the options**
d. Assessment for more facts

Complementary Bodywork Systems

Massage terms and treatments typically found on spa menus

Hydrotherapy tub and associated treatments
    MEDICAL CONCERNS
    TYPES OF TUB TREATMENTS
    CLEANING THE TUB AND ROOM
    FOIL AND PLASTIC FOR WRAPPING
      Foil
      Plastic

Aromatherapy
    HOW ESSENTIAL OILS WORK

The massage practitioner's responsibilities in the spa environment

SUMMARY

▼INSTRUCTOROBJECTIVES

1. Present the physiologic mechanisms of complementary bodywork systems.
2. Identify similarities in bodywork methods.
3. Compare wellness massage with medical massage.
4. Identify the overlap in technical skills among the various systems, and integrate concepts of the styles into the therapeutic massage system.
5. Explain the general effects of hot- and cold-water applications.
6. Discuss and demonstrate how to incorporate simple hydrotherapy methods into the massage setting.
7. Explain the general effects of lymphatic and circulation enhancement massage. For more information on the systems and pathologic conditions, see Chapter 11 in *Mosby's Essential Sciences for Therapeutic Massage: Anatomy, Physiology, Biomechanics, and Pathology,* second edition.
8. Demonstrate how to incorporate the principles of lymphatic and circulation massage into the general massage session. Also see Chapter 11 in *Mosby's Essential Sciences.*
9. Explain the physiologic benefits of foot and hand massage.
10. Explain how to incorporate the principles of reflexology into the general massage session.
11. Demonstrate how to modify existing massage methods to address more specifically the connective tissue. Tissue repair and connective tissue are also discussed in Chapters 1, 2, 8, and 9 in *Mosby's Essential Sciences.*
12. Explain the principles of deep transverse friction massage.
13. Describe a trigger point.
14. Demonstrate how to locate a trigger point. Also see Chapter 9 in *Mosby's Essential Sciences* for individual muscle discussion, as well s localized and referred pain patterns of trigger points.
15. Demonstrate two methods to massage a trigger point.
16. Explain the basic physiology of acupuncture points and the effects of acupressure. Ancient healing practices and acupuncture can be reviewed in *Mosby's Essential Sciences* for additional information.
17. Demonstrate how to locate an acupuncture point.
18. Demonstrate how to use simple methods to stimulate or sedate acupuncture points.
19. Discuss introductory Ayurvedic terminology and similarities in massage methods.
20. Review the 12 main meridians and their pathologic conditions. Use the pathology appendix in *Mosby's Essential Sciences* to discuss the possible meridian that is hindered.
21. Explain the basic theory of polarity therapy.
22. Demonstrate how to incorporate the principles of polarity therapy into the massage session.
23. Discuss how the information in this text and the science text can be applied in the spa environment.
24. Explore with the students various directions of interest for further study.

CHAPTER SUMMARY

This chapter introduces systems of structured touch other than therapeutic massage. The individual systems can be categorized as follows:

- Eastern and Asian thought involving vital energy, chakras, meridians, and points
- Reflex systems such as hydrotherapy and reflexology
- Energetic systems such as polarity
- Structural systems such as Rolfing shiatsu, myofascial release, and cranial sacral approaches
- Spa concepts and how the massage therapist functions within this environment

Suggestions for incorporating simple methods for each of the approaches are included in the chapter.

CHAPTER HIGHLIGHTS AND POINTS FOR DISCUSSION

Discuss the following statement: You can apply pressure, lift and stretch tissue, rock the body, stroke the skin, entrain the rhythms, move the joints, generate tissue repair by creating therapeutic inflammation, stimulate reflex responses, soothe the energy field, and provide interpersonal and professional support, compassion, and acceptance of the client. All of the bodywork systems, including therapeutic massage—regardless of the theoretical, cultural, and historical base—are built on this same foundation.

Discuss the following statement: Expertise in any bodywork system consists of *quality assessment* to make *effective decisions* about the *application of treatment* to provide the *service that benefits* the client.

Massage methods can be used in various forms of health care, rehabilitative, or athletic massage. For the massage professional to use the methods in a more specific way, additional training is needed, especially pathophysiology, pharmacology, and medical treatment protocols.

When dealing with medical conditions and working within the health care environment, the massage therapist will find that the methods (massage manipulations and techniques) described in Chapter 9 or any of the various methods described in the text do not change. What differs is the condition of the person receiving the massage. Additional education does not usually pertain to learning new methods but rather learning how to choose and use methods with clients who have various complex pathologic conditions.

Discuss and demonstrate various spa menu applications and their relevance to integrations with therapeutic massage. Discuss the importance and need for ongoing education, and explain what information is presented during continuing education.

Hydrotherapy

Hydrotherapy is a separate and distinct form of therapy that combines well with massage and is used extensively in the spa and sport environments. Water can be used in many different ways, depending on the health needs and condition of the client and the facilities available for therapy.

Water can relax or stimulate, anesthetize, and reduce or increase circulation. Water works naturally and is nonallergenic, tissue tolerant, inexpensive, and readily available.

Water's three forms (liquid, steam, and ice) allow for its use in a variety of temperatures.

Discuss applications of hydrotherapy appropriate to the massage setting.

Lymphatic and Blood Circulation

Many variations and styles of massage are used to stimulate lymphatic and blood circulation.

All massage stimulates the circulation and lymph movement, but structuring a massage to focus on this system is a specific therapeutic intervention.

The pressure that massage provides mimics the compressive forces of movement and respiration to stimulate circulation and lymphatic flow.

Discuss the anatomy and physiology of these bodywork systems in relation to the application of the methods described in this text and *Mosby's Essential Sciences*, Chapter 11. Point out that methodology is based on interaction with physiologic processes and that specific methodology is developed to best interact with the anatomy and physiology. Demonstrate the methods while connecting them to the applicable anatomy and physiology.

Reflexology

In the bodywork community, *reflexology* refers to the stimulation of areas beneath the skin to improve the function of the whole body or of specific body areas that are away from the site of the stimulation.

Reflexology applies the stimulus/reflex principle to healing the body. The medical definition of reflexology is "the study of reflexes." *Reflexotherapy* is the treatment by manipulation or other means applied to an area away from the disorder.

Discuss the reflexive nature of massage and why stimulation of the hands and feet is an effective way to stimulate reflexive body systems.

Connective Tissue Systems

Connective tissue systems range from the very subtle, light work of cranial-sacral and fascial release concepts to the very mechanical deep transverse frictioning of Cyriax's syndrome. These styles of bodywork are often called *deep-tissue massage, soft-tissue manipulation,* or *myofascial release.* The basic connective tissue approach consists of mechanically softening the tissue through pressure, pulling, movement, and stretch on the tissues, which allows them to rehydrate and become more pliable. Also see Chapters 8 and 9 in *Mosby's Essential Sciences.*

If dysfunction occurs in the fascial network, efficiency of the body is compromised, requiring an increase in energy expenditure to achieve functioning ability. Fascial dysfunction is seldom simple and almost always multidimensional, often encompassing body/emotion phenomena because body armoring is an effective coping strategy. Introducing corrective intervention is a therapeutic change process akin to remodeling a house (Chapter 5 of the textbook). If the person is unable to respond effectively to a change process, management approaches can be offered, but effects pertain more to symptom management than structural change.

Discuss and demonstrate the various connective tissue applications. Review the therapeutic change process presented in Chapter 5 of the textbook and relate it to connective tissue methods.

Trigger Point Therapy

Trigger point therapy is one of many useful techniques for treating myofascial problems. Perpetuating factors to the development of trigger points are reflexive, mechanical, and systemic. See the individual muscles in Chapter 9 in *Mosby's Essential Sciences* for the trigger point locations and referred pain patterns.

Only the muscles that can actually be treated at the same visit should be examined. Palpating for trigger points can irritate their referred pain activity, thus only areas intended for treatment should be palpated.

All of the basic neuromuscular techniques, including the muscle energy techniques (Chapter 9 in the textbook), will deal effectively with trigger points *if* the hyperirritable area within a muscle is hyperstimulated and then lengthened and the connective tissue in the area is softened and stretched.

Discuss and demonstrate the various trigger point approaches.

Asian Bodywork Methods

This section presented in this textbook is based on a limited part of the total Asian medicine system. Taking pieces from the totality being expressed in the Tao is problematic. Western science has lifted technique from this simple yet complex, all-encompassing system. Technique separated from its theoretical basis is often less effective. Although technique can stimulate physiologic functions, it cannot support the human experience. The unity of body, mind, and spirit revolves around our energy for life. In Asian life theory, our life force is called *Chi* when all pathways, or meridians, are balanced.

Acupuncture is defined as the stimulation of certain points with needles inserted along the meridians (channels) and *AhShi* (meaning "ouch") points outside the meridians. *AhShi* and traditional acupuncture points have a high degree of correlation to trigger points.

Acupressure is a modified version of acupuncture that substitutes pressure for needle insertion. Meridians seem to be energy flows from nerve tracks in the tissue and are located in the fascial grooves.

The Asian perspective considers body functions in terms of balance between complementary forces. Yin and yang are representations of this concept.

Chinese medical thinking is based on the relationship of the human being with nature. The five elements of nature become a basis for the examination, diagnosis, and treatment to support health and relieve disease. The five elements are wood, fire, earth, metal, and water.

Discuss the various Asian medicine principles that influence massage therapy.

Demonstrate the methods that effectively integrate with therapeutic massage.

Ayurveda

Ayurveda is a system of health and medicine that grew from roots in East India. Ayurveda means life knowledge or right living. The principle is grounded as a body-mind-spirit system in the Vedic scriptures. The tridosha theory is unique to this system. A dosha is a body chemical pattern. When the doshas combine, they constitute the nature of every living organism. The three doshas are *Vata* or wind, *Pitta* or bile, and *Kapha* or mucus. These three doshas combine to form five elements (similar to Asian theory) of ether, air, fire, water, and earth.

The points connected with this system are called *marmas*. Approximately 100 of these points can be found, and they are concentrated at the junctions of muscles, vessels, ligaments, bones, and joints. Marmas have a strong correlation to common trigger points and the location of the traditional meridians (see Figure 11-12 in this book).

Chakras are seven centers of the Prana located along the spinal column and interrelated with the nervous system and endocrine glands.

Discuss, compare, and contrast the Ayurvedic system with the other systems presented in the text.

Polarity

Polarity is a holistic health practice that encompasses some of the theory base of Asian medicine and Ayurveda. Entrainment is one of the most plausible of the physiologic responses to explain the benefits of polarity. Some polarity techniques involve rocking motions; therefore all physiologic benefits of rocking as discussed in Chapter 9 would apply. Gentle stimulation by polarity methods to the joint receptors generates reflex response to the associated muscles.

When the professional has no attachment to the outcome for his or her own individual sense of achievement, the methods become "free" to influence the experience of the client.

Polarity therapy does not treat illness or disease; it affects the body (life) energy, which flows in invisible electromagnetic currents through the body's organs and tissues. The purpose of polarity therapy is to stimulate the energy that is inactive in a diseased body part.

Discuss and demonstrate the application of polarity, both as a technique and as a way of being and interacting with clients in the therapeutic massage setting.

The Spa Environment

Discuss the following points.

Therapeutic massage complements the spa environment in many ways, particularly the use of complementary bodywork modalities found in spa menus. Assessment and treatment plan development in the spa setting may need to be modified for the client receiving a single massage without ongoing care. Condition management and palliative care may also be appropriate in the spa environment with emphasis on pampering and pleasure. Using various procedures and essential oils requires knowledge to achieve expected outcomes.

Hydrotherapy is effectively integrated in the spa environment. Current trends for the spa are to evolve into an integrated health experience. This shift will increase the necessary and required skills of the massage practitioner to support a retention client base.

MULTIPLE-CHOICE TEST BANK

_____ 1. The effects of water are primarily:
   a. Mechanical
   b. Placebo
   c. Reflexive
   d. Palliative

_____ 2. P.R.I.C.E. as a first-aid treatment:
   a. Increases recovery time and muscle spasm
   b. Is appropriate for most soft-tissue injuries
   c. Stands for recovery, ice, circulation, and exercise
   d. Is best applied 24 hours after the injury

_____ 3. When doing specific lymph drain massage:
   a. The client may feel ill for 48 hours after the session.
   b. No additional training is required to work with lymphedema.
   c. It is not a specific therapeutic intervention.
   d. The therapist uses deep sustained pressure.

_____ 4. Circulatory massage:
   a. Should be done only on people with cardiovascular problems
   b. For venous circulation begins at the fingertips
   c. Is indicated on varicose veins
   d. Over arteries uses compression

_____ 5. In reflexology, the big toe represents the:
   a. Foot
   b. Lungs
   c. Head and neck
   d. Hara

_____ 6. With connective tissue work:
   a. Stretching, pulling, and applying pressure may provide benefits.
   b. Overstretching tissues at joints will cause joint stability.
   c. The work is best done without any other methods.
   d. Using any form of muscle energy methods before stretching is unnecessary.

_____ 7. Cross-fiber frictioning:
   a. Is used mainly in cranial release methods
   b. Should be localized to one specific area
   c. Requires lubrication to reduce the adhesions
   d. Should last no more than 3 seconds

_____ 8. A trigger point is found in a muscle:
   a. And can be aggravated only by physical stress or trauma
   b. And is considered a large area of hypotonicity
   c. That attaches to the skeletal system
   d. That is only of the phasic type

_____ 9. Yin and yang:
   a. Reflect only the body, not the mind
   b. Work only on the reproductive systems of the male or female
   c. Pair meridians so that yin meridians are on the left and yang meridians are on the right
   d. Reflect sympathetic and parasympathetic activities

_____ 10. Polarity:
   a. Encompasses some of the theory base of Asian medicine and Ayurveda
   b. Uses rocking methods but does not focus movement at the joints
   c. Is a specific method for treating disease
   d. Works independent of the energy system of the body

_____ 11. A client has mild edema in the lower legs from a long plane flight the previous day. Which of the following is an appropriate treatment plan?
   a. Short light gliding strokes focused on the legs. Compression to the sole of the foot. Active and passive joint movement for the ankle, knee and hip. Place the leg above the heart.
   b. Compression to the legs focused on the medial side form proximal to distal. Muscle energy and lengthening combined with stretching in the area of the most accumulation of fluid.
   c. Deep gliding strokes from proximal to distal on the legs. Place the legs above the heart. Limit movement to encourage drainage.
   d. Superficial and deep compression along the vessels in the lateral leg. Active resistive joint movement combined with shaking.

_____ 12. A client injured the right shoulder 3 years ago. Assessment indicates decreased mobility of the skin surrounding the shoulder coupled with a painful but normal range of motion. Which is the best treatment option for this client?
   a. Deep transverse friction
   b. Superficial myofascial release
   c. Compression
   d. Lymphatic drainage

_____ 13. Which is a correct way to sedate a hyperactive acupuncture point?
   a. Tap the point.
   b. Vibrate the point.
   c. Apply sustained pressure on the point.
   d. Stimulate the meridian containing the point.

_____ 14. A client has a cough and nasal mucus. Diarrhea and intestinal cramping are also present. The large intestine meridian is tender to the touch. Which other meridian that is part of the metal element is directly involved?
   a. Pericardium
   b. Lung
   c. Bladder
   d. Heart

_____ 15. When treating trigger points:
   a. Direct pressure methods and squeeze methods should be used first.
   b. Positional release with lengthening is the first application method.
   c. Connective tissue stretching needs to accompany muscle energy application.
   d. Lengthening of the tissue housing the trigger point is only effective with a local tissue stretch.

Serving Special Populations

▼CONTENTOUTLINE

PREGNANCY
  The first trimester
  The second trimester
  The third trimester
  Disorders of pregnancy
  Labor
  Recommendations for massage during pregnancy
TERMINAL ILLNESS
SUMMARY

▼ INSTRUCTOR OBJECTIVES

1. Discuss how to develop a massage environment to best serve individuals with special needs.
2. Demonstrate the communication skills that are important when working with a client who has special needs.
3. Present data concerning additional training and information about massage for people with special needs.
4. Discuss how to integrate therapeutic massage into the health care environment.
5. Define abuse.
6. Explain state-dependent memory.
7. Discuss criteria to help the student recognize dissociation.
8. List the elements needed in additional training to work specifically with abuse issues.
9. Demonstrate how to respond resourcefully if a client responds emotionally during a massage.
10. List the experts in care and training for athletes and how massage supports athletes.
11. Explain the three types of restorative massage.
12. Explain the concept of event sport massage.
13. List the components that are necessary for additional sports massage training.
14. Identify when breast massage is appropriate. Review breast cancer in Chapter 11 in *Mosby's Essential Sciences for Therapeutic Massage: Anatomy, Physiology, Biomechanics, and Pathology,* second edition.
15. Discuss ethical principles to determine when breast massage is performed.
16. Demonstrate how to apply general massage methods to ease growing pains.
17. Discuss how to train family members in massage techniques for use at home.
18. Explain the basic cause of chronic illness.
19. Explain the difference between acute illness and chronic illness.
20. Assist the student in developing realistic expectations for working with people who have chronic illnesses.
21. Discuss benefits of massage for older adults.
22. Discuss the possible need for fee and time adjustments when working with older adults.
23. Explain the importance of the first year of life for an infant.

24. Explain the importance of organized sensory stimulation for infants.
25. Demonstrate how to teach parents to massage their infants.
26. Discuss the importance of a confident touch when working with infants.
27. Explain the importance of supervision in the health care setting.
28. Describe written and verbal communication necessary for working in the health care environment.
29. List special considerations for working with clients who are undergoing medical treatment either in the health care environment or home health care setting.
30. Discuss and demonstrate how to communicate more effectively with people who have a physical disability.
31. Discuss how to adjust the massage environment to better support individuals with physical disabilities.
32. Present criteria to help a student become aware of subtle discrimination.
33. Discuss the importance of verifying informed consent when working with individuals with a psychologic disability.
34. Discuss how massage may support other psychologic interventions.
35. Explain the importance of prenatal care.
36. Describe the three basic stages of pregnancy. Additional information regarding pregnancy can be found in Chapter 12 in *Mosby's Essential Sciences* and the pathology appendix in the same book.
37. Demonstrate a general massage session to meet the needs of a pregnant woman.
38. Demonstrate how to teach a support person basic massage methods to use during labor.
39. Discuss the dying process. Explain the importance of comfort measures.

CHAPTER SUMMARY

This chapter examines ways in which the massage professional can respect and help people who need special consideration. The intent of the information is to help the massage professional focus the benefits of therapeutic massage for clients with specific needs such as athletes to compassion during terminal illness. Integration of therapeutic massage into the health care environment is also presented, because many who have special needs also require the support of diverse health care professionals. Each section offers a general description of the special situation, the application for massage, and directions for obtaining further training and information. The massage therapist who desires to focus his or her professional skills to best meet the specific needs of a person or environment will continue to seek out training and information that is pertinent to the therapeutic needs of each client. In many instances, the knowledge base required to provide massage to multiple populations becomes too extensive, and specializing becomes necessary. The wise professional recognizes when less intervention is more appropriate. This recognition requires much learning, great skill, and patiently developed empathy to hold someone's hand therapeutically.

CHAPTER HIGHLIGHTS AND POINTS FOR DISCUSSION

Abuse

Discuss the following points.

When people are abused, survival mechanisms take many forms, such as dissociation, hypervigilance, aggressive behavior, learning to "disappear," low self-esteem, and withdrawal. Post-traumatic stress disorder is common. These patterns may generalize into many life situations.

State-dependent memory is encoded in the brain in a manner that includes the position, emotion, chemicals, nervous system activation, and all other combined physiology affecting the internal functions of a person at the time the experience happened. Later, when the physical and emotional states change, the memory may be vague or forgotten. State-dependent memory functions in all life experiences. When someone gets ready to hit a baseball or drive a car, he or she will assume the appropriate position, and the body will remember. During trauma, this mechanism locks in all the factors that coincide with the experience. As time passes, this repressed memory may be triggered by any one of the sensations and physiologic factors involved in the state-dependent memory.

Some life experiences that may affect a person in a manner similar to abuse are illness, medical procedures, hospitalization, accidents, or other trauma. The success of the individual's coping skills will depend on the type of support received during and soon after the traumatic event, as well as the dynamics surrounding the situation.

The touch of the massage therapist may remind the body of the abuse or trauma.

The massage practitioner should never remove a coping mechanism for a client or imply guilt for using it when a purpose is being served. The decision to deal actively with an abusive history requires commitment and time from the client. Professional help and support groups are often needed. People who do not want to recover their memories of abuse must also be considered. A difference exists between the *reenactment* of abuse and an *integration* process that may result from the physical triggers that massage produces. Reenactment involves reliving the event as if it were happening again right at that moment. Integration is involved more with remem-

bering the event while being able to remain in the present moment with an awareness of the difference between then and now so as to bring some sort of resolution to the event.

Reenactment does not necessarily provide the awareness and understanding that are necessary to integrate the physical response and emotional feelings into the client's experience in an empowering way. The massage professional needs to be aware of the potential for causing possible harm to the client by deliberately triggering a reenactment response. Without the additional and necessary support of qualified counselors and other support personnel to provide for an integration process, a reenactment is undesirable.

If a client responds during the massage by crying, shaking, panicking, becoming agitated or fearful, or demonstrating another emotional pattern, the massage professional should be quiet and let the person experience the emotion. The practitioner must not interfere with the person's experience by interjecting suggestions.

IMPORTANT NOTE: **Not all emotional responses during massage indicate a past abuse situation. The emotional pattern may be a reflection of current stressors or life events. The response may be chemical in origin. Caution students not to prematurely interpret the response but instead remain open to many possibilities.**

Athletes

Discuss the following points.

Athletes are people who participate in sports, either as amateurs or professionals. The athlete trains the nervous system and muscles to perform in a specific way. The activity often involves the repetitive use of one group of muscles more than others, which can result in hypertrophy, changes in strength patterns, changes in connective tissue formation, and compensation patterns in the rest of the body.

Joint injuries are also common among athletes because of the repetition of training and performing. Also see Chapter 8 in *Mosby's Essential Sciences.*

The physical activity of an athlete goes beyond fitness and is based on performance . Although physical activity is necessary for an athlete, fitness is necessary for everyone's wellness. It concept is explained in Chapter 13 of the textbook.

Massage can be beneficial for athletes if the professional performing the massage understands the biomechanics that the sport requires. If not, massage can impair optimal function in the athletic performance. Because of the intense physical activity involved in sports, an athlete may be more prone to injury.

Common Sport Injury

One of the most important aspects of sport massage is to assist the athlete in achieving and maintaining peak performance, as well as to support healing of injuries. Any massage professional should recognize common sport injury and refer to the appropriate medical profession. Once a diagnosis is determined and the rehabilitation plan is developed, the massage professional can support the athlete with general massage application and appropriate methods to enhance the healing process.

The experts for athletes are the sports medicine physician, physical therapist, athletic trainer, exercise physiologist, and sports psychologist. Any type of massage before a competition must be given carefully.

The classifications for massage given to athletes are:
- Restorative massage
- Recovery massage
- Remedial massage
- Rehabilitation massage

Before the event, warm-up massage is a stimulating, superficial, fast-paced, rhythmic massage lasting 10 to 15 minutes.

Intercompetition massage, given during breaks in the event, concentrates on muscles that are being used or are about to be used. The techniques are short, light, and relaxing.

After the event, warm-down massage can reduce muscle tension, minimize swelling and soreness, encourage relaxation, and reduce recuperation time.

For athletes, regular massage allows the body to function with less restriction and accelerates recovery time. Most athletes require varying depths of pressure from light to very deep. Therefore effective body mechanics by the massage practitioner is essential. Working with athletes can be demanding. Athletes' schedule may be erratic, and their body changes almost daily in response to training, competition, or injury. Athletes can become dependent on massage, thus commitment by the massage professional is necessary. Many specialized training programs for sports massage are available. If the massage professional intends to work with athletes, additional training must be pursued. Such training should include the physiologic and psychologic functions of an athlete; overuse and repetitive use syndromes; the biomechanics of specific sports; the use of cryotherapy, ice massage, and other hydrotherapy methods; injury repair and rehabilitation; and education in training regimens.

NOTE: **Any person involved in an activity or profession that requires repetitive movement, such as the factory worker, mail carrier, waiter or waitress, dentist, musician, or massage practitioner, can be assisted using massage applications that are similar to those of the athlete.**

Breast Massage

Discuss the following points.

The massage of the female breast is a controversial issue. A conservative approach is taken in this textbook.

Breast massage can be appropriate for certain conditions such as fibrosis and scar tissue development resulting from surgery of various types.

If breast massage for a specific condition is deemed appropriate by a health care professional and referral is made, the following recommendations are suggested:
- Work with specific informed consent for breast massage.
- Work with another professional in the room, just as a gynecologist has a female nurse present when giving examinations. If this precaution is not possible, male therapists should consider referring a female client to a female therapist.
- Careful draping is provided. Do not expose the entire breast unless absolutely necessary. Do not expose both breasts.
- Work gently, professionally, and confidently.
- Avoid the nipple area.

Ethical consideration for breast massage must be considered. Discuss the ethical consideration for breast massage, especially in the wellness setting, with relaxation and pleasure goals as outcomes.

Children

Discuss the following points.

Providing massage services for children is not much different than providing services for adults. Because children and adolescents may have shorter attention spans than adults, a 30-minute massage is usually sufficient. The practitioner never works with children and adolescents without parental or guardian supervision.

Discuss the importance of supervision when working with children.

Chronic Illness

Discuss the following points.

Chronic illness is defined as a disease, injury, or syndrome showing little change or slow progression. Dealing with chronic illness is difficult for the person who has the affliction, for the physician and health care team, and for the massage therapist.

Working with chronic illness does not often produce measurable results. People with chronic illnesses are usually under the care of a physician and may be taking medications. The massage professional must work closely with the medical professionals who are involved to understand the effects of the various medical treatments and medications.

The massage professional who wishes to work with the chronically ill needs to have realistic expectations. Instead of developing a massage approach to bring about a cure for the illness, which is out of the scope of massage practice, the focus should be on helping the client feel better for a little while. The benefits of massage may provide enough relief for clients to be able to find the necessary inner resources to deal with the effects of chronic illness constructively, increasing the quality of their lives and the lives of people around them.

Discuss the possibility of burnout for the professional when dealing with clients with chronic illness. Discuss the unique benefits that massage offers these clients and how these benefits may affect the total treatment program.

Older Adults

Discuss the following points.

People in their advanced years can benefit greatly from massage. Although the methods of massage are not different when working with elderly patients, these clients do present specific challenges.

Many older adults take multiple medications, are often depressed, and experience periods of insomnia or disrupted sleep patterns. Many older adults are alone. The interaction with a massage therapist can provide both physical and emotional stimulation for this population.

If a person does not have adequate cognitive functioning skills, as in cases of dementia caused either by the aging process or by medications taken for other conditions, he or she will be unable to give informed consent for the massage. The guardian, physician, or other health care professional will then need to intervene to give the necessary permission to provide massage.

Discuss the value of massage for older adults and obstacles for providing massage to this population.

Infants

Discuss the following points.

Infants cannot give informed consent; therefore parents must provide this permission and remain present during any professional interaction with the infant.

Research by Dr. Tiffany Fields and her associates shows that premature infants who have been massaged fare much better than those who have not.

Parents should be taught to massage their own infants. Consideration must be given to a shorter massage time (between 15 and 30 minutes), to the smaller, still developing anatomy, and to the needs of the parents as they learn to communicate with their infants through touch.

Refer to Chapter 4 and discuss the research of Dr. Tiffany Field at the Touch Research Institute.

Medical Intervention and Support

Discuss the following points.

Working with clients in a health care environment, such as a hospital, rehabilitation center, extended care facility, or mental health facility, presents special situations.

The massage professional will be functioning as part of a health care team, following the objectives of a comprehensively designed treatment plan.

The entire plan is supervised, usually by a physician. Most communication occurs in written form via treatment orders and charting. Standard Precautions and other sanitation procedures must be followed precisely. Various medications and their interaction with the effects of the massage must be considered.

Effects from medical testing procedures or preparation for testing procedures will affect massage intervention.

The challenge of working in the health care environment is not how to work with the specific client, but rather how to interact effectively with the health care professionals serving the client. The skill levels presented in the text are sufficient to provide this type of care if the professional is qualified to work in the complex health care environment. The skills necessary to function in the health care environment include education in:

- Clinical reasoning
- Problem solving
- Justifications for treatment
- The ability to set qualifiable and quantifiable goals
- Medical terminology
- Pathology
- Various medical tests and procedures
- Medications
- Assessment
- Developing treatment plans
- Analyzing the effectiveness of the methodsused
- Charting
- The ability to communicate information effectively effectively

Discuss the previous skill levels in terms of the student's present competency levels.

Identify areas that may require additional education.

Physically Challenged Individuals

Discuss the following points.

People with physical impairments can benefit from massage just as any other individual can. The client's body may develop a compensation pattern for the disability. The person with a disability should be treated the same as anyone else. The right of individuals to choose the kind of help they need must be respected.

A therapist must never presume to know, understand, or anticipate a client's need. *It is important to ask!*

All massage facilities must be barrier free. Commercial buildings are usually required by law to have a barrier-free access, elevators, and restroom facilities for the physically handicapped. Discuss important accommodations to serve individuals with physical challenges.

Psychologically Challenged Individuals

This section considers:
- Addictions
- Chemical imbalances in the brain
- Developmental disabilities
- Learning disabilities
- Mood disorders
- Post-traumatic stress disorder

Discuss the following points.

Again, the actual massage approach is really not different. The important factor is who is receiving the massage. People who wish to work with clients with psychologic challenges will need additional training to be able to understand the physiology and psychology of the various disorders and the challenges these clients face.

Understanding psychotropic pharmacology is important because massage affects the body in ways similar to these medications. A psychologist or psychiatrist should closely supervise this type of work.

General stress-reduction massage may moderate the mood through its influence on the autonomic nervous system. The type of massage given can be adjusted to be a little more stimulating or a little more relaxing.

Massage affects the brain chemicals by encouraging the release of serotonin, dopamine, and endorphins, as well as other neurotransmitters and hormones that alter mood. Massage has a strong normalizing effect on the autonomic nervous system and can support other interventions for psychiatric disorders.

Discuss the benefits of combining massage with other mental health interventions.

Pregnancy

Discuss the following points.

Pregnancy is not an illness; it is a natural event. Prenatal care is needed to make sure that proper nutrition is provided for the mother, that the pregnancy is progressing normally, and that any potential problems are identified early.

Pregnancy is divided into three distinct segments: the first, second, and third trimesters. A woman who is pregnant is undergoing extensive physical and emotional changes during each of these stages.

Unless specific circumstances or complications exist, massage for pregnant women should be a general massage. Do not massage vigorously or extremely deep, overstretch, or massage the abdomen other than superficial stroking. Avoid massage on the inside of the ankle because a reflex point is located there that stimulates uterine contractions. Watch for fever, edema, varicose veins, and severe mood swings. After the birth, postpartum depression can become a serious problem for some women. Refer the client with these conditions immediately to the client's physician.

Discuss positioning and any other factors necessary to support prenatal massage.

Terminal Illness

Discuss the following points.

The experts in situations of terminal illness are the dedicated hospice nurses and staff who treat death with dignity.

For the massage practitioner to work successfully with individuals dealing with a terminal illness, the practitioner must be aware of his or her personal feelings about death.

Massage can offer the terminally ill patient temporary comfort. Being bedridden and immobile is painful. Massage can distract the sensory perception, provides continued human contact, and can give caregivers something useful, rewarding, and positive to do for their loved one who is dying.

Massage can become an important stress-reduction method and a means of support for family members and caregivers.

Discuss the commitment necessary to work with terminally ill patients and their caregivers and family.

MULTIPLE-CHOICE TEST BANK

_____ 1. The gentle, caring touch of a massage professional:
- a. Causes the client to create dissociative coping mechanisms
- **b. May still remind a client of an abusive or traumatic situation**
- c. Will never create an uneasy feeling in a client
- d. Is always more effective than counseling

_____ 2. When a client cries, shakes, or shows emotion during the massage:
- a. Stop the massage immediately and remove your hands.
- **b. Ask if you should continue the massage.**
- c. Talk until the person becomes calm.
- d. Ask the client to talk to you about the memory or situation.

_____ 3. Postevent massage:
- a. Is a vigorous 1-hour massage
- b. Requires lubricants to be most effective
- **c. Is a quick-paced, superficial routine**
- d. Includes trigger point and connective tissue work

_____ 4. Having realistic expectations when working with people with chronic illness includes:
   a. Understanding that not getting worse may be an improvement
   b. Knowing that deterioration will stop
   c. Knowing that massage can cure many illnesses
   d. Realizing that palliative care is inappropriate

_____ 5. In many people over the age of 70:
   a. The bones usually become more flexible.
   b. The skin is thinner, and circulation is not as efficient.
   c. Injury repair is increased.
   d. The aging process causes skin to thicken and circulation to increase.

_____ 6. Infant massage:
   a. Calms the parent as much as the child
   b. Should take between 30 and 45 minutes daily
   c. Does not require informed consent
   d. Always calms the infant

_____ 7. When a person has a physical disability:
   a. Speak loudly and slowly.
   b. Additional assistance will always be needed.
   c. He or she cannot provide informed consent.
   d. Ask what assistance is needed.

_____ 8. During pregnancy:
   a. Morning sickness is most common in the third trimester.
   b. The connective tissue shortens and thickens.
   c. Position during the massage is a consideration.
   d. Working on the legs does not involve any precautions.

_____ 9. Hospice staff and family members of the terminally ill patient:
   a. Do not need massage because the focus is on the person with the illness
   b. Should not be trained to do massage on the person with the illness
   c. Should allow only licensed massage therapists to do the massage
   d. May welcome a caring massage professional

_____ 10. When providing massage to a person with special needs:
   a. Rubber gloves must be worn.
   b. Keep the session private, and do not include family members.
   c. Remember to be caring and respectful, just as you would with any other client.
   d. Focus specifically on the special need.

_____ 11. A massage therapist has just started a job at a medical family practice center. The center deals with many clients who exhibit stress-related symptoms. Which of the following professional skills will the massage therapist need to perfect?
   a. Muscle energy methods
   b. Restorative massage
   c. Charting and record keeping
   d. Lymphatic drainage

_____ 12. Which of the following would be contraindicated for hot hydrotherapy treatment?
   a. An athlete
   b. A referred client from a psychologist
   c. A woman in her first trimester of pregnancy
   d. Someone with a neck impingement

_____ 13. A college football player is seeking massage as part of a healing program for an injured knee that required surgical intervention. The athletic trainer is supervising the massage. The massage consists of general full-body massage that addresses any developing compensation resulting from the gait change while the knee is healing. Specific applications of kneading and myofascial release are being used to maintain pliability in the soft tissue of the upper and lower leg. What type of massage is being preformed?
   a. Postevent massage
   b. Recovery massage
   c. Remedial massage
   d. Rehabilitation massage

_____ 14. When doing the necessary assessments and paperwork before working with an athlete at an event, the massage professional notices that the athlete has hot skin, rapid pulse, shallow breathing, and is very flushed. What health condition might the athlete be experiencing?
   a. Anxiety over the sports event
   b. Muscle cramps
   c. Heatstroke
   d. Indigestion

CHAPTER

13

Wellness Education

▼ INSTRUCTOR**OBJECTIVES**

1. Identify the basic components of a wellness program.
2. Provide guidance in locating resources to develop a wellness program.
3. Demonstrate methods used to provide general wellness guidelines to clients.

CHAPTER SUMMARY

The purpose of this chapter is to educate the massage professional about the general concepts of wellness. Wellness is living life in a simple, gentle, respectful way—for ourselves and with others. Wellness is the result of the healing that takes place on multiple levels when we take care of ourselves, which then extends to caring for others and the planet in general. Wellness is peace within. Sharing that peace in simple ways, consistently with respect and compassion, can support the wellness of us all and peace for our world. This chapter examines the basic guidelines that are necessary for building a wellness program. Enough information is provided to give some direction in developing and implementing a wellness plan.

CHAPTER HIGHLIGHTS AND POINTS FOR DISCUSSION

Wellness Programs

Wellness programs can be built around these factors:

Body:
- Nutrition
- Light and dark exposure
- Sleep
- Breathing
- Movement and fitness
- Sensory stimulation

Mind:
- Relationships with self and others
- Communication
- Beliefs
- Intellectual stimulation

Spirit:
- Purpose
- Connection
- Faith
- Hope
- Love

Discuss the importance of each wellness factor and how each one supports the others.

We are considered *well* when body, mind, and spirit are in ideal balance. We are not well when imbalance exists and when balance cannot be restored.

Massage practitioners need to remember that although massage is wonderful, it addresses only a part of the person. Wellness is about the whole person.

Discuss when and how massage is most supportive in a wellness program.

Wellness has a domino effect. Making a simple alteration in lifestyle will have a chain reaction through your entire life.

Making a change to wellness takes determination.

Stress is our response to any demand on the body or mind to respond, adapt, or alter.

Discuss the stress response. Refer to textbook Chapters 4 and 5, as well as Chapter 2, in *Mosby's Essential Sciences for Therapeutic Massage: Anatomy, Physiology, Biomechanics, and Pathology,* second edition.

Before any wellness program can be developed, a person needs to at least "explore thyself." The next step is to analyze and explore the stressors that we all encounter in our daily lives.

The three major elements of stress are (1) the stressor itself, (2) the defensive measures, and (3) the mechanisms for surrender.

The massage professional will recognize that the signs of stress result from fluctuations in the autonomic nerv-ous system and resulting endogenous chemical shifts. Also see Chapter 5 in *Mosby's Essential Sciences.*

Discuss the signs of stress and relate them to risk factors presented in Chapter 5.

Today, many of the demands placed on us are outside the design of the body. Wellness often revolves around simplification of the lifestyle. Simplification requires choices, boundaries, discipline, and letting go in many dimensions.

Loss heals through grieving. Grief is a physiologic response that includes stimulation of the sympathetic autonomic nervous system.

Wellness training requires an extensive amount of information about diet, exercise, lifestyle, and behavior patterns. The massage practitioner must seek out people with experience to provide this information. Many professionals can help us with specific therapeutic interventions as the wellness program is developed. Physicians, counselors, other health care providers, educators, and religious advisors all have an important part to play in helping us become well again or maintain our wellness.

Discuss the role the massage professional plays as part of a wellness support team.

Exercise and stretching programs are important parts of any wellness program because they provide the activity that our body was designed to have. Exercise has become an essential purpose unto itself. Fitness programs need to be appropriate; exercise systems and stretching programs must be modified to fit the individual. Massage is an excellent way to support flexibility programs, especially if the methods used address both the elasticity and the pliability of the soft tissue.

Appropriate exercise is necessary for wellness and varies for each individual. Because the components of an exercise program can be accomplished in a variety of ways, people can engage in many activities that support health. Massage professionals serve and encounter various clients, from infants to older adults, from the athlete to the business professional. Students must learn about the basics of a fitness program as described in the chapter to provide both general education about wellness and to complement various fitness programs.

MULTIPLE-CHOICE TEST BANK

_____ 1. Massage is an important part of a wellness program because it:
   a. Supports body balance and connects with another human being
   b. Is defined as a step-by-step process
   c. Follows general concepts
   d. Does not address "vertical illness"

_____ 2. One important factor to know about stress is that it:
   a. Is always a destructive breakdown
   b. Is always outside of our control
   c. Can be used to support resourceful change
   d. Is not helped by honesty with ourselves

_____ 3. When warning signs of stress appear:
   a. It is an indication of a genetic risk factor.
   b. It is helpful to divert the body's attention to something else.
   c. People respond in a predictable way.
   d. The most vulnerable part of the physiology will continue to function well.

_____ 4. Communicating effectively is best considered as:
   a. An objective matter
   b. The presentation of information and personal interpretation
   c. One of the most difficult challenges for human beings
   d. A minor part of wellness

_____ 5. Redirecting a disease pattern toward a more healing pattern:
   a. Takes a combination of only a few lifestyle changes
   b. Takes many major lifestyle changes
   c. Takes resources that are beyond the means of most human beings
   d. Cannot be achieved from wellness information

_____ 6. A sound wellness program needs to:
   a. Rely on medical professionals
   b. Be based on a particular self-help program
   c. Be complex and all encompassing
   d. Balance intuition and research

_____ 7. Massage practice can be compared with wellness because:
   a. Both are based on complex theory.
   b. Both need to be built on fundamentals.
   c. Each approach works for everyone.
   d. Both are to be limited in the scope study.

_____ 8. A wellness program needs to:
   a. Remain consistent, regardless of circumstances
   b. Rely on support in only one area of function
   c. Change as we change
   d. Evolve specifically through nutritional change

_____ 9. Eating affects:
   a. Mood
   b. Only tissue repair
   c. Primarily regeneration
   d. Specifically sleep disorders

_____ 10. Breathing patterns:
   a. Are inappropriate for mediation
   b. Can alter mood and behavior
   c. Depend only on the quality of air
   d. Are not affected by tight muscles

_____ 11. Aerobic exercise training is an exercise program focused on increasing what?
   a. Immune system and body strength
   b. Hand coordination and fitness
   c. Fitness and endurance
   d. Eye coordination and dance abilities

_____ 12. An exercise program consists of three components. Two of them are warm-up and aerobic exercise. What is the third component?
   a. Cool down
   b. Hydration
   c. Adequate footwear
   d. Adaptation

Business Considerations for a Career in Therapeutic Massage

▼CONTENTOUTLINE

▼INSTRUCTOROBJECTIVES

1. Assist the student in determining his or her personal motivation for developing a therapeutic massage career.
2. List the pros and cons for independent status or employee status.
3. Present information to help the student understand the commitment required to develop a massage therapy business.
4. Present information to help the student understand the importance of motivation for successful business development.
5. Discuss criteria to help a student determine a suitable target market and a sustaining retention client base.
6. Discuss strengths and weaknesses that will add to or detract from developing a successful business.
7. Discuss methods to prevent "burnout."
8. Discuss development of a 5-year business plan.
9. Describe a resume.
10. Describe business goals.
11. Discuss start-up costs.
12. Explore marketing strategies and advertising materials for a massage business.
13. Discuss a word-of-mouth marketing plan.
14. Develop criteria that are necessary for the informational brochure, business card, and media story.
15. Explore fee structures for therapeutic massage services.
16. Investigate whether third-party insurance reimbursement is available or appropriate for the practice of therapeutic massage.
17. Present criteria for negotiating lease agreements based on either a percentage of gross receipts or a flat fee.
18. Discuss average overhead expenses and yearly income.
19. Present a step-by-step procedure to set up business-management practices.
20. Demonstrate how to set up business files. Present various business-management and record-keeping systems.

CHAPTER SUMMARY

This chapter presents specific information for people who are wishing to develop a massage business. The chapter does not attempt to be a small business management text. The information presented will be unique to therapeutic massage and sufficient to guide the student to additional learning. The chapter shares the experience of being a massage professional. Completing all of the activities in the chapter helps the student develop a business plan and decide whether being self-employed or an employee would better serve him or her.

CHAPTER HIGHLIGHTS AND POINTS FOR DISCUSSION

Being successfully self-employed requires an entrepreneurial spirit. Self-employed people must be self-starters with a broad range of professional and business skills.

Discuss the entrepreneurial spirit. Discuss whether the entrepreneurial spirit is necessary to build a successful massage career.

The profession has seen a steady increase in available jobs and career opportunities in the more traditional employee market in which the massage practitioner works for an individual or company at an hourly wage or salary.

Discuss what has changed to support more opportunities in the employee sector for massage professionals.

To succeed at anything, the individual must be motivated. The components of motivation are listed. Discuss each of the following:
* Knowing thyself
* Following your dream
* Experience
* Self-concept
* Believing in your product
* Providing a quality product

Discuss the following points.
* *Burnout* occurs when energy is used faster than it is restored.
* A resume is a professional and personal data sheet.
* Having a plan when setting up a business is important. A *mission statement* expresses the intent of the business plan. To develop a mission statement, answer this question: What will be the main focus of my business?
* After the "big picture" concepts of the business plan are in place, smaller steps to implement the plans are identified. These steps are the goals.
* Start-up costs are the initial expenses required to begin a business.
* Successful massage professionals are commonly found operating in many different formats.

Posing the following questions helps the student narrow and develop a target market for a therapeutic massage career:
* Where do you plan to work?
* Who lives or works within a 30-minute drive of the location?
* What type of massage or bodywork do you enjoy giving?
* Who are the people you want to help most?
* How are you going to reach these potential clients?
* When do you want to be available to do massage?

Marketing is the advertising and other promotional activities that are required to sell a product or service. *Word-of-mouth* is the best form of advertising.

A regular base clientele of approximately 100 is sufficient to support a thriving therapeutic massage business. Talking to 2000 people to find 100 clients may be necessary. The most successful massage practices are based on retention and repeat visits.

The main marketing obstacle to personal-service wellness massage is convincing the public that regular massage is beneficial in a total lifestyle program that is focused on managing stress and striving for wellness.

The brochure is the primary tool to educate the public and potential clients concerning the services being offered. Any written material or advertising must answer these questions for potential clients:
* Who? (you)
* What? (therapeutic massage)
* Where? (address and phone number)
* When? (appointment times)
* How? (they can reach you by phone)

Another concern for the client is how much the massage will cost. Charging what a massage is worth in time value is important. This practice is especially important for the regular client who will need to budget massage costs and justifying the expenditure.

Insurance companies that pay for wellness-oriented personal-service therapeutic massage is uncommon. If the massage therapist is an employee of a licensed medical professional or managed care corporation, which has access to insurance billing codes, and is working under direct supervision, the massage services may be covered by insurance. Payment by the client for services rendered is the most dependable income base.

Management includes all the activities that are required to maintain a business, particularly record keeping and financial disbursement. The KISS principle (i.e., keep it simple and specific) is an excellent concept to help organize the details of business practices.

All business receipts must be saved and filed. Copies of all important documents should be stored in a different location from the originals. Everything must be dated, and no verbal contracts should be made. Information should be organized monthly on a spreadsheet so that when the time comes for the tax preparer to file the business and personal taxes, everything can be verified. This so-called "paper trail" is important for a properly run business, and it must be established.

Discuss each of the points on the following checklist for business setup:

- Obtaining a license
  - a. Business license
  - b. Professional practice license or ordinance
- Choosing a business location
- Determining business legal structure
- Obtaining a DBA designation
- Arranging for registration for taxes such as sales taxes
- Arranging for insurance
- Establishing business banking accounts
- Setting up investments
- Keeping records
- Providing a client-practitioner agreement and policy statement

MULTIPLE-CHOICE TEST BANK

_____ 1. Motivation:
   a. Is offensive to clients and must be limited
   b. Begins once the market is defined
   c. Is only needed by self-employed massage therapists
   d. Is an internal drive that helps accomplish goals

_____ 2. The business portion of massage:
   a. Is organized and disciplined
   b. Cannot be handled by the average person
   c. Does not require any professional assistance
   d. Does not qualify for assistance from the small business association

_____ 3. A resume:
   a. Should list only work experience that relates to massage
   b. Is a personal and professional summary
   c. Is developed after the business plan
   d. Should list only education and not work experience

_____ 4. Start-up costs:
   a. Are the costs for the first month of operation
   b. Are any of the initial costs of beginning a business
   c. Should include business cards and brochures but not furniture and equipment
   d. Do not include refundable rent deposits

_____ 5. When marketing:
   a. Remember that newspaper advertising is inexpensive.
   b. Giving free talks and demonstrations is unwise.
   c. Remember that a brochure is a costly investment that has little return for the investment.
   d. Remember that a happy client may be the best advertisement.

_____ 6. Insurance reimbursement:
   a. Requires minimum paperwork
   b. Is commonly received for massage services
   c. May be possible if the massage therapist is an employee of a licensed medical professional who can bill for massage
   d. Is approved if the massage therapist submits the proper code

_____ 7. Business operations show that:
   a. One half of the income is usually spent on overhead costs.
   b. Most massage practitioners are employees of other therapists.
   c. Renting space is more costly than buying a building.
   d. Subcontractors can be told when to work and what to wear.

_____ 8. Being a massage employee:
   a. Is less desirable than being self-employed because you have to answer to an employer.
   b. Can be a great career opportunity without the responsibility of all business operations
   c. Means that you are less motivated than the self-employed person
   d. Will likely result in less income than self-employment

_____ 9. Taxes:
   a. Do not have to be paid by independent contractors
   b. Usually work out to one twentieth of business income
   c. Need to be set aside annually
   d. Must be paid whether the massage therapist is an employee or is self-employed

_____ 10. Business records:
   a. Need to be saved for only 1 year
   b. Should be kept in a clear, simple, organized manner
   c. Do not need to be kept for verbal agreements
   d. Are valid only if approved by a certified public accountant

_____ 11. Gross income minus expenses equals:
   a. Deductions
   b. Deposits
   c. Net income
   d. A draw

_____ 12. Expenses that are used to begin new business operations are called:
   a. Business plans
   b. Reimbursements
   c. Investments
   d. Start-up costs

Case Studies

▼ CONTENT OUTLINE

▼ CHAPTER SUMMARY

Each of the case studies in this chapter should challenge your students to continue to develop clinical reasoning skills and to perfect assessment and technical therapeutic massage skills.

This chapter integrates the information from both this textbook and the student's science studies, such as the content covered in Mosby's Essential Sciences. Competency in therapeutic massage practice is reflected in the ability to understand the content of science studies and how to put the information into practical application with individual clients.

The 20 case studies in this chapter cover the most common outcome goals of clients. The listed case studies cover at least 80% of the common conditions seen by massage professionals in day and destination spas and wellness, health, fitness, sport, and medical settings.

▼ INSTRUCTOR OBJECTIVE

1. Encourage your students to use this chapter as a self-study tool.

▼ STUDENT OBJECTIVES

After completing this chapter, the student will be able to perform the following:

1. Use critical reasoning to integrate the information from science studies and this text to complete a comprehensive history, assessment, and care/treatment plan.
2. Write comprehensive case studies.
3. Analyze care/treatment plans, and offer and justify alternate approaches to care.

Appendix:
Competencies for
Therapeutic Massage

A rubric is a method of measuring competencies in a progressive process. Rubric levels begin with 1, which is the least competent and reflects the beginner; they end with 6, which reflects full competency. Students in programs of 500 contact hours should expect to achieve a minimum of level 3 competencies, whereas those in longer-running programs can strive for level 5 or level 6 proficiency. Students are able to self-assess using the criteria presented. Instructing staff members can use rubric levels as a way of measuring the progression of students and as a guide for examinations. Each individual program may have a slightly different focus, depending on the philosophy of the school or according to state or local regulations. The rubric pattern presented can be easily modified to accommodate these special situations. The "Practical Examination Performance Evaluation" in this appendix on page 86 should be used in conjunction with the following rubric.

COMPETENCIES FOR THERAPEUTIC MASSAGE

Entry-level, 500 to 750 hours, 25 to 35 credits factored at 15 hours per one credit of lecture and 30 hours per one credit of laboratory or practicum

RUBRIC: MEASURING COMPETENCIES IN A PROGRESSIVE PROCESS

CRITERIA I: Demonstrates the ability to perform massage methods in an ergonomically correct manner using a massage table, chair, or mat (body mechanics).

Level 1: Relies on hand and arm strength with little use of leverage, forearms, or modified positioning of client. Bends elbows, does not maintain weight on appropriate foot, and does not align the body to prevent torsion of the shoulders, pelvis, and knees. Is routinely on top of stroke instead of behind it. Cannot maintain a stable body position but collapses head, shoulders, and core muscles.

Level 2: Uses leverage with proper position of the client but not consistently. Tends to overuse hand and arm strength with repetitive motion at the shoulder joint instead of entire body movement. Recognizes ineffective body mechanics but is unable to self-correct. Works to the middle range of pressures but is unable to modify to either extremely light pressure or heavy pressure. Struggles to maintain a stable body position.

Level 3: Is able to use positioning of the client to maximize leverage but continues to overuse hands. Bends elbows, uses repetitive movement, and so forth but is beginning to self-correct. Can modify to light pressure but is unable to provide maximal pressures. Maintains a stable and aligned body position. Uses self-massage and stretching measures before, during, and after sessions.

CRITERIA II: Understands the application and can explain the physiologic outcome of all massage manipulations and techniques as described in Chapter 9 of *Mosby's Fundamentals of Therapeutic Massage.*

Level 1: Is able to locate information in textbook but is unable to apply textbook information in practical application.

Level 2: Interprets textbook information concerning physiologic outcomes and demonstrates methods but struggles to correlate to practical applications as part of a total massage session.

Level 3: Is able to describe the application of a method in terms that are accurate but different from that of the textbook. Is able to correlate to various practical applications during massage. Correlates all applications to physiologic outcomes. Provides simple applications for teaching self-help methods to clients.

CRITERIA III: Applies and modifies each of the following standard massage methods as described in Chapter 9 of *Mosby's Fundamentals of Therapeutic Massage:* gliding stroke, kneading, compression vibration, shaking, rocking, percussion, and friction.

Level 1: Is able to perform each method but is unable to perform all methods in all four basic positions (prone, supine, lateral recumbent, and seated) with variations in intensity, duration, direction, speed, and rhythm in all body areas.

Level 2: Interprets textbook information and demonstrates methods but struggles to correlate to practical applications as part of a total massage session.

Level 3: Performs all methods on all body areas in all four basic positions without using the textbooks. Is beginning to adjust application to appropriate depth, intensity, duration, direction, speed, and rhythm based on client goals.

CRITERIA IV: Able to apply and modify each of the massage techniques and methods (found in *Mosby's Fundamentals of Therapeutic Massage,* Chapter 9) in four basic positions: prone, supine, lateral/recumbent, and seated.

Level 1: Is able to perform each method but unable to perform all methods in all positions with variations in intensity, duration, direction, speed, and rhythm in all body areas.

Level 2: Interprets textbook information concerning physiological outcomes and demonstrates methods but struggles to correlate to practical applications as part of a total massage session.

Level 3: Performs all methods on all body areas in all four basic positions using textbooks. Is beginning to adjust application to appropriate depth, intensity, duration, direction, speed, and rhythm based on client goals.

RUBRIC: MEASURING COMPETENCIES IN A PROGRESSIVE PROCESS—cont'd

Level 4: Maximizes leverage through positioning the client. Uses body weight to apply pressure and easily uses supported hands, forearms, knees and foot to accomplish methods. Occasionally overuses hand or arm strength with repetitive motions but self-corrects quickly. Maintains stable alignment and body position, changing position frequently.

Level 5: Self-corrects body mechanics. Easily recognizes use of muscle action instead of leverage to apply pressure. Makes appropriate choices for using the hand, arm, knee, or foot to accomplish task. Continues to struggle to provide and sustain delivery of maximal pressure.

Level 6: Demonstrates full and competent use of body, using varied positioning of the client and body leverage methods to apply a full range of pressure depths to all body areas. Is able to self-massage and stretch self to counteract any muscle tension from the massage application.

Level 4: Is able to describe the application of a method with variations and modifications inclusive of, as well as different from, the textbook criteria. Thinks in terms of choosing methods based on client goals and physiologic outcomes.

Level 5: Is able to compare and contrast various methods in terms of applications, practical use, and overlapping applications. Continually chooses appropriate methods based on outcomes. Provides ongoing appropriate education and description to client. Is able to discuss various self-help applications, teaching each as self-help methods. Is able to use description of methods, applications, and physiologic outcomes to justify treatment plans and communicate with health or fitness professionals.

Level 6: Is able to teach the applications in a client self-help method, specifically focusing on client outcomes. Comprehends, easily combines, and modifies method described based on multimodel treatment plans.

Level 4: Performs all methods on all body areas in all four basic positions. Adjusts depth, intensity, duration, direction, speed, and rhythm appropriately to client outcomes.

Level 5: Is able to flow effectively with all methods, using a variety of positioning and choosing depth, intensity, duration, direction, speed, and rhythm based on client outcomes.

Level 6: Is able to combine various methods—positioning, intensity, duration, direction, and speed—to achieve specific treatment goal, justifying each application.

Level 4: Performs all methods on all body areas in all four basic positions. Adjusts depth, intensity, duration, direction, speed, and rhythm appropriately to client outcomes.

Level 5: Is able to integrate all methods effectively, using a variety of positioning and choosing depth, intensity, duration, direction, speed, and rhythm based on client outcomes.

Level 6: Combines various methods—positioning, intensity, duration, direction, and speed—to achieve specific treatment goal, justifying each application.

Continued

RUBRIC: MEASURING COMPETENCIES IN A PROGRESSIVE PROCESS—cont'd

CRITERIA V: Can apply and modify each of the massage methods and techniques in the areas of neck, shoulder, arm, wrist/hand, thorax anterior, thorax posterior, abdomen, lumbar, gluteus, hip, leg, ankle, foot.

Level 1: Is able to perform each method but is unable to perform all methods in all positions with variations in depth, intensity, duration, direction, speed, and rhythm in all body areas.

Level 2: Interprets textbook information concerning physiologic outcomes and demonstrates methods but struggles to correlate to practical applications as part of a total massage session.

Level 3: Performs all methods on all body areas in all four basic positions using textbooks. Is beginning to adjust application to appropriate depth, intensity, duration, direction, speed, and rhythm based on client goals.

CRITERIA VI: Student performs and integrates passive and active joint movement during assessment and therapeutic session applications for the following: neck (cervical and capital), shoulder, elbow, wrist, finger and thumb, vertebral column, hip, knee, ankle, toes.

Level 1: Is able to perform with the use of the textbooks but is not confident with positioning, body mechanics, and stabilization, or how to incorporate assessment application into a massage session.

Level 2: Is able to perform with the use of textbooks and incorporates effective body mechanics, stabilization, and simple integration into the assessment process. Is able to perform in all four basic positions (prone, supine, lateral recumbent, and seated).

Level 3: Is able to perform effectively in relationship to assessment procedures. Integrates smoothly into the massage session, choosing the best positioning of the client for execution of the movement pattern and the best position for body mechanics and stabilization.

CRITERIA VII: Able to perform muscle-energy techniques on the muscles below as listed in Chapter 9 of *Mosby's Fundamentals of Therapeutic Massage* and Chapter 9 of *Mosby's Essential Sciences for Therapeutic Massage: Anatomy, Physiology, Biomechanics, and Pathology*. Is also able to incorporate application of various mechanical forces, lengthening, trigger point therapy, stretching, and myofascial or structural approaches for the following: occipitofrontalis, masseter, temporalis, sternocleidomastoid, longus capitis, scalenus anterior, scalenus medius, scalenus posterior, splenius capitis, cervicis, erector spinae group (sacrospinalis), spinalis (thoracis, cervicis, and capitis), longissimus (thoracis, cervicis, and capitis), iliocostalis (lumborum, thoracis, and cervicis), the transversospinalis group, semispinalis (thoracis, cervicis, and capitis), intertransversarii (lumborum, thoracis, and cervicis), interspinales, the suboccipital muscles, rectus capitis posterior major, rectus capitis posterior minor, oblique capitis superior, oblique capitis inferior, diaphragm, external intercostals, internal intercostals, innermost intercostals, transversus thoracis, quadratus lumborum, psoas major, psoas minor, iliacus transversus abdominis, rectus abdominis, internal oblique, external oblique, trapezius, rhomboid major, rhomboid minor, levator scapula, pectoralis minor, serratus anterior, supraspinatus, infraspinatus, teres minor, subscapularis, deltoid, pectoralis major, latissimus dorsi, teres major, coracobrachialis, biceps brachii, brachialis, brachioradialis, pronator teres, triceps brachii, anconeus, supinator, pronator quadratus, flexor carpi radialis, palmaris longus, flexor carpi ulnaris, flexor digitorum superficialis, flexor, digitorum profundus, flexor pollicis longus, extensor carpi radialis longus, extensor carpi radialis brevis, extensor digitorum, extensor digiti minimi, extensor carpi ulnaris, abductor pollicis longus, extensor pollicis brevis, extensor pollicis longus, extensor indicis, opponens pollicis, abductor pollicis brevis, flexor pollicis brevis, opponens digiti minimi, abductor digiti minimi, flexor digiti minimi (brevis), adductor pollicis, interossei palmares, interossei dorsales, lumbricales, gluteus maximus, gluteus medius, gluteus minimus, tensor fasciae latae, piriformis, obturator internus, obturator externus, quadratus femoris, gemellus superior, gemellus inferior, hamstring group, semimembranosus, semitendinosus, biceps femoris, pectineus, adductor brevis, adductor longus, adductor magnus, gracilis, sartorius, quadriceps femoris group, rectus femoris, vastus lateralis, vastus intermedius, vastus medialis, tibialis anterior, extensor digitorum longus, extensor hallucis longus, peroneus tertius, peroneus longus, peroneus brevis, popliteus, tibialis posterior, flexor digitorum longus, flexor hallucis longus, plantaris, soleus, gastrocnemius, extensor digitorum brevis, abductor hallucis, flexor digitorum brevis, abductor digiti minimi, quadratus plantae, lumbricales, flexor hallucis brevis, adductor hallucis, flexor digiti minimi brevis, interossei plantares.

Level 1: Is able to perform with the use of the textbooks but is not confident with positioning, body mechanics, and stabilization, or how to incorporate assessment into a massage session.

Level 2: Is able to perform with the use of textbooks and incorporates effective body mechanics, stabilization, and simple integration into the assessment process. Is able to perform in all four basic positions (prone, supine, lateral recumbent, and seated).

Level 3: Is able to perform effectively in relationship to assessment procedures. Integrates smoothly into the massage session, choosing the best positioning of the client for execution of the movement pattern position for body mechanics and stabilization. Can identify superficial, intermediate muscles but struggles to access and address deeper muscles.

RUBRIC: MEASURING COMPETENCIES IN A PROGRESSIVE PROCESS—cont'd

Level 4: Performs all methods on all body areas in all four basic positions. Adjusts depth, intensity, duration, direction, speed, and rhythm appropriately to client outcomes.

Level 5: Is able to integrate all methods on all body areas using a variety of positioning and choosing depth, intensity, duration, direction, speed, and rhythm based on client outcomes.

Level 6: Combines various methods to address all body areas—positioning, intensity, depth, duration, direction, and speed—to achieve specific treatment goal, justifying each application.

Level 4: Actively uses joint movement during preassessment and postassessment and as positioning for lengthening and stretching procedures.

Level 5: Solves problems using joint movement methods to assess and analyze information to determine primary and compensation patterns. Integrates smoothly as part of assessment and intervention procedures.

Level 6: Actively translates and integrates joint movement with preassessment and postassessment. Uses joint movement actively in muscle energy lengthening and stretching procedures.

Level 4: Actively uses joint movement during pre- and postassessment and as positioning for muscles during lengthening and stretching procedures. Is able to apply mechanical forces to all layers of muscle, superficial to deep.

Level 5: Actively integrates muscle isolations and muscle testing into assessment procedures to identify and apply appropriate intervention methods.

Level 6: Is able to treat shortened, weakened, and compensation patterns with full integration of methods. Is able to address connective-tissue shortening and fibrosis with multiple methods, justifying all interventions to treatment plan.

Continued

RUBRIC: MEASURING COMPETENCIES IN A PROGRESSIVE PROCESS—cont'd

CRITERIA VIII: Demonstrates appropriate sanitation and Universal precaution procedures, as well as equipment and premise safety procedures.

Level 1: Is unable to perform safety and sanitation measures consistently using textbook support.

Level 2: Performs safety and sanitation measures with textbook support.

Level 3: Performs safety and sanitation measures without textbook support but not always consistently.

CRITERIA IX: Demonstrates, explains, and modifies draping procedures in four basic positions: prone, supine, lateral recumbent, and seated.

Level 1: Is unable to perform draping methods in four basic positions.

Level 2: Using textbook diagrams, is able to perform draping methods in four basic positions, including abdominal draping, gluteal draping, and chest draping.

Level 3: Performs basic draping methods for all body areas without textbook support.

CRITERIA X: Assesses clients both subjectively (by obtaining a client history and client outcome goals) and objectively (through a physical assessment using observation, palpation, and basic differential testing). Identifies indications and therapeutic goals appropriate for entry-level therapeutic massage or determines cautions and contraindications for therapeutic massage and need for referral.

Analyzes assessment information to develop therapeutic massage applications appropriate for entry-level training in terms of intensity (depth of pressure and drag), direction, speed, rhythm, frequency, and duration. Demonstrates appropriate choice of methods, including gliding strokes, kneading, compression, vibration, shaking, rocking, percussion, friction, joint movement, muscle energy techniques, lengthening, and stretching to achieve client outcome goals.

Level 1: Is able to complete all segments of client history and physical assessment form but is unable to analyze data effectively.

Level 2: Completes a basic assessment, including muscle testing, and effectively analyzes data for indications and contraindications or need for referral.

Level 3: Is able to collect and analyze assessment information for application of various methods to achieve client goals.

CRITERIA XI: Demonstrates charting, record-keeping, and justification procedures. Develops appropriate care and treatment plans using clinical-reasoning/problem-solving and justification procedures.

Intake procedures include informed consent, client history, physical assessment, care and treatment plan, and permission to release information.

Ongoing record keeping includes session charting, updating history and physical assessment, modifying and updating treatment plans, and keeping financial records.

Special record keeping includes writing narrative reports for health care providers and developing interventions or treatment plans for reimbursement.

Level 1: Is unable to complete all forms and categories. Is unable to record information to the appropriate form or to identify proper location on the form, even with textbook support.

Level 2: Is able to complete forms using textbook support but is unable to consistently apply clinical-reasoning methodology to analyze information. Is able to communicate with client concerning informed consent but is unable to justify effectively the record-keeping process.

Level 3: Is able to complete record-keeping process without textbook support but is unable to consistently use the clinical-reasoning methods as an approach to record-keeping procedures.

Level 4: Constantly maintains safety and sanitation methods. Accommodates all safety and sanitation measures to unique situations.

Level 5: Performs in health care systems based on standard precautions, following directives.

Level 6: Constantly maintains and is able to accommodate safety and sanitation methods regardless of environmental situation.

Level 4: Is able to modify textbook draping methods in all four positions for all body areas as necessary for any unique circumstance.

Level 5: Is able to improvise draping procedures to accommodate various special circumstances.

Level 6: Is able to drape effectively in any circumstance.

Level 4: Is able to collect and analyze assessment data for treatment plan development and justification for using methods to achieve client goals.

Level 5: Completes a comprehensive history and physical assessment, analyzing data for interactive compensation pattern, treatment plan development, and modification of application of methods.

Level 6: Is able to integrate assessment data into a comprehensive treatment plan and justification of all methods used, including appropriate variation of methods to address specific circumstances and goals.

Level 4: Consistently integrates clinical-reasoning and justification procedures into record-keeping methodology.

Level 5: Generates treatment plans from assessment data justified through using clinical-reasoning methodology.

Level 6: Is able to maintain ongoing record-keeping procedures, consistently using clinical reasoning methods. Justifies treatment plans and completes narrative reports as necessary.

Continued

RUBRIC: MEASURING COMPETENCIES IN A PROGRESSIVE PROCESS—cont'd

CRITERIA XII: Describes behaviors relating to profession ethics, scope of practice, and standards of practice. During massage, demonstrates professional and ethical decision making using a model of clinical reasoning and problem solving. Describes and demonstrates methods of self-monitoring of technical skills to include body mechanics and method applications and maintains appropriate boundaries to support the integrity of the therapeutic relationship. Describes and demonstrates empathic, respectful, and professional communication skills.

Level 1: Can recite textbook data but does not understand ethical application. Processes feedback constructively but forms a reactive and emotional stance.

Level 2: Understands concepts of scope of practice, standards of practice, boundary and communication issues, and ethical dilemmas but does not use the decision-making model to resolve issues. Hesitates to use effective communication to provide feedback. Is willing to self-monitor behavior and accept constructive and corrective feedback both from peers and staff.

Level 3: Actively uses the ethical decision-making model to analyze professional behaviors of self and clients. Is able to identify difficulties but is not always confident on how to solve issues. Uses communication skills to address issues but occasionally avoids conflict. Understands the dynamics of peer support and how to use the decision-making model in a peer support dialogue.

RUBRIC: MEASURING COMPETENCIES IN A PROGRESSIVE PROCESS—cont'd

Level 4: Anticipates ethical dilemmas and uses ethical decision-making and communication skills to resolve issues before they become problematic. Seeks peer support and mentoring as an ongoing process, especially when dealing with conflict.

Level 5: Responds appropriately to complex client-practitioner- health care professional dynamics in a proactive and professional way. Deals with conflict objectively, using the ethical decision-making model and communication skills.

Level 6: Actively self-monitors behavior, making appropriate adjustments and seeking peer support and mentoring assistance when necessary. No longer avoids conflict but instead remains process oriented.

PRACTICAL EXAMINATION
PERFORMANCE EVALUATION

This form consists of a front and back side. The entire form must be reviewed by the student and an instructor/evaluator and signed by both. Test Coordinator is to forward to the administration office within 5 days of examination date.

Date: _____   Instructor/Evaluator: _____

Student Name: _____   Circle One: Evaluation   1   2   3   4

INSTRUCTIONS:

1. Refer to competency document to score criteria for criteria I-XII.
2. Circle the appropriate score for each criteria.
3. Add up score and divide by 12 at the end of practical examination to receive competency level.

CRITERIA I

Demonstrates the ability to perform massage methods in an ergonomically correct manner using a massage table, chair, or mat. (body mechanics).

Score = 1, 1.25, 1.50, 1.75, 2, 2.25, 2.50, 2.75, 3, 3.25, 3.50, 3.75, 4, 4.25, 4.50, 4.75, 5, 5.25, 5.50, 5.75, 6

CRITERIA II

Understands the application and can explain the physiologic outcome of all massage manipulations and techniques as described in Chapter 9 of *Mosby's Fundamentals of Therapeutic Massage*.

Score = 1, 1.25, 1.50, 1.75, 2, 2.25, 2.50, 2.75, 3, 3.25, 3.50, 3.75, 4, 4.25, 4.50, 4.75, 5, 5.25, 5.50, 5.75, 6

CRITERIA III

Applies and modifies each of the following standard massage methods as described in Chapter 9 of *Mosby's Fundamentals of Therapeutic Massage*: gliding stroke, kneading, compression, vibration, shaking, rocking, percussion, friction.

Score = 1, 1.25, 1.50, 1.75, 2, 2.25, 2.50, 2.75, 3, 3.25, 3.50, 3.75, 4, 4.25, 4.50, 4.75, 5, 5.25, 5.50, 5.75, 6

CRITERIA IV

Able to apply and modify each of the massage techniques and methods in four basic positions: prone, supine, lateral/recumbent, seated.

Score = 1, 1.25, 1.50, 1.75, 2, 2.25, 2.50, 2.75, 3, 3.25, 3.50, 3.75, 4, 4.25, 4.50, 4.75, 5, 5.25, 5.50, 5.75, 6

CRITERIA V

Can apply and modify each of the massage methods and techniques in the areas of neck, shoulder, arm, wrist/hand, thorax anterior, thorax posterior, abdomen, lumbar, gluteus, hip, leg, ankle, foot.

Score = 1, 1.25, 1.50, 1.75, 2, 2.25, 2.50, 2.75, 3, 3.25, 3.50, 3.75, 4, 4.25, 4.50, 4.75, 5, 5.25, 5.50, 5.75, 6

CRITERIA VI

Student performs and integrates passive and active joint movement during assessment and session applications for the following: neck (cervical and capital), shoulder, elbow, wrist, finger and thumb, vertebral column, hip, knee, ankle, toes.

Score = 1, 1.25, 1.50, 1.75, 2, 2.25, 2.50, 2.75, 3, 3.25, 3.50, 3.75, 4, 4.25, 4.50, 4.75, 5, 5.25, 5.50, 5.75, 6

CRITERIA VII

Able to perform muscle energy techniques (as listed in Chapter 9 of *Mosby's Fundamentals of Therapeutic Massage*) on the muscles listed in the competency document and Chapter 9 of *Mosby's Essential Sciences for Therapeutic Massage.* Is also able to incorporate lengthening, trigger point therapy, stretching, and myofascial/structural approaches for those same muscles.

Score = 1, 1.25, 1.50, 1.75, 2, 2.25, 2.50, 2.75, 3, 3.25, 3.50, 3.75, 4, 4.25, 4.50, 4.75, 5, 5.25, 5.50, 5.75, 6

CRITERIA VIII

Demonstrates appropriate sanitation and standard precaution procedures, as well as equipment and premise safety procedures.

Score = 1, 1.25, 1.50, 1.75, 2, 2.25, 2.50, 2.75, 3, 3.25, 3.50, 3.75, 4, 4.25, 4.50, 4.75, 5, 5.25, 5.50, 5.75, 6

CRITERIA IX

Demonstrates, explains, and modifies draping procedures in four basic positions: prone, supine, lateral recumbent, seated.

Score = 1, 1.25, 1.50, 1.75, 2, 2.25, 2.50, 2.75, 3, 3.25, 3.50, 3.75, 4, 4.25, 4.50, 4.75, 5, 5.25, 5.50, 5.75, 6

CRITERIA X

Assesses clients both subjectively (by obtaining a client history and client outcome goals) and objectively (through a physical assessment using observation, palpation, and basic differential testing). Identifies indications and therapeutic goals appropriate for entry-level therapeutic massage and/or determines cautions and contraindications for therapeutic massage and need for referral.

Score = 1, 1.25, 1.50, 1.75, 2, 2.25, 2.50, 2.75, 3, 3.25, 3.50, 3.75, 4, 4.25, 4.50, 4.75, 5, 5.25, 5.50, 5.75, 6

CRITERIA XI

Demonstrates charting, record-keeping, and justification procedures. Develops appropriate care/treatment plans using clinical-reasoning/problem-solving and justification procedures. *Intake procedures to include:* informed consent, client history, physical assessment, care/treatment plan, permission to release information. *Ongoing record keeping to include:* session charting, updating history and physical assessment, modifying and updating treatment plans, keeping financial records. *Special record keeping to include:* writing narrative reports for health care providers and developing interventions/treatment plans for reimbursement.

Score = 1, 1.25, 1.50, 1.75, 2, 2.25, 2.50, 2.75, 3, 3.25, 3.50, 3.75, 4, 4.25, 4.50, 4.75, 5, 5.25, 5.50, 5.75, 6

CRITERIA XII

Will describe behaviors relating to professional ethics, scope of practice, and standards of practice. During massage, demonstrates professional and ethical decision making using a model of clinical-reasoning/problem solving. Describes and demonstrates methods of self-monitoring of technical skills to include body mechanics and method applications and maintains appropriate boundaries to support the integrity of the therapeutic relationship. Describes and demonstrates empathic, respectful, and professional communication skills.

Score = 1, 1.25, 1.50, 1.75, 2, 2.25, 2.50, 2.75, 3, 3.25, 3.50, 3.75, 4, 4.25, 4.50, 4.75, 5, 5.25, 5.50, 5.75, 6

I have read my evaluation report and the student advising comments and have discussed these with an instructor. I understand that all fails must be reported to the Director of Education.

Student signature: _____

Instructor/Evaluator signature: _____ Date: _____

Note: A copy of this report is given to the student. Original should go to the Administration Office.

Transparency Masters

The following transparency masters can be used in the classroom. We have included figure numbers as they appear in the book, as well as transparency master numbers, titles, and credit lines as needed.

TM 1   Major Chakras
TM 2   Historical Timeline
TM 3   Scope of Therapeutic Massage Practice
TM 4   Divisions of the Nervous System
TM 5   Acupuncture Points, Motor Points, and Cutaneous Nerves
TM 6   Major Nerve Plexuses
TM 7   Benefits of Massage
TM 8   Referred Pain
TM 9   Endangerment Sites
TM 10 Body Mechanics for Compressive Force
TM 11 Body Mechanics for Petrissage and Stretching
TM 12 Flow Pattern in the Colon
TM 13 Joint Movements
TM 14 Midline Balance Point
TM 15 Efficient Gait Position
TM 16 Rocking Movement of the Sacral Iliac Joint
TM 17 Fascial Sheaths
TM 18 Quadrants and Movement Segments
TM 19 Postural Influences on Muscle Patterns
TM 20 Strokes for Facilitating Lymphatic Flow
TM 21 Compression for Increasing Arterial Flow
TM 22 Effleurage Strokes for Facilitating Venous Flow
TM 23 Generalized Reflexology Chart
TM 24 Common Trigger Points
TM 25 Typical Locations of Meridians
TM 26 Relationship between the Five Elements and the Organs
TM 27 Vertical Electromagnetic Currents
TM 28 Brain Wave Currents
TM 29 Characteristics, Clinical Signs, and Interventions of Stages of Tissue Healing

Transparency Master 1

Major Chakras (Fig. 1-3)

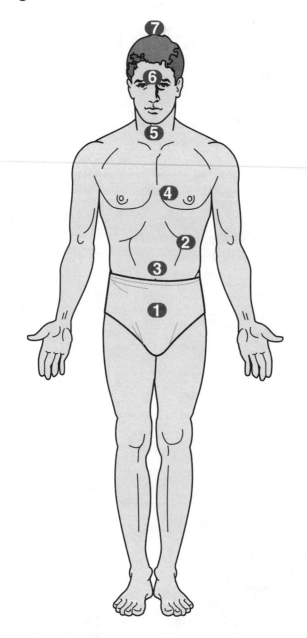

	English Name	Situation
1	Root or basic chakra	At the base of the spine
2	Spleen or splenic chakra	Over the spleen
3	Navel or umbilical chakra	At the navel, over the solar plexus
4	Heart or cardiac chakra	Over the heart
5	Throat or laryngeal chakra	At the front of the throat
6	Brow or frontal chakra	In the space between the eyebrows
7	Crown or coronal chakra	On the top of the head

Transparency Master 2
Historical Timeline (Fig. 1-4)

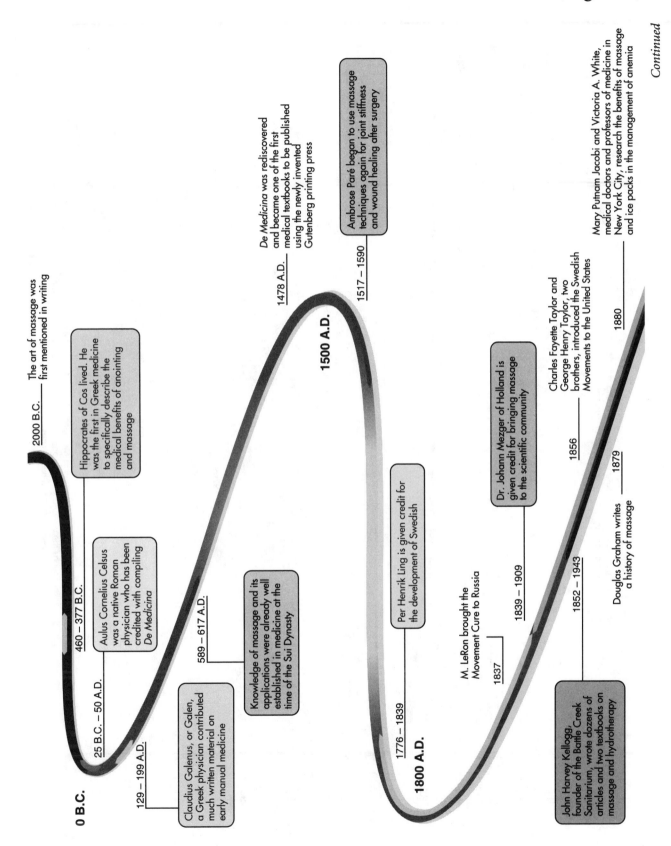

Continued

2000 B.C. — The art of massage was first mentioned in writing

460 – 377 B.C. — Hippocrates of Cos lived. He was the first in Greek medicine to specifically describe the medical benefits of anointing and massage

25 B.C. – 50 A.D. — Aulus Cornelius Celsus was a native Roman physician who has been credited with compiling *De Medicina*

0 B.C.

129 – 199 A.D. — Claudius Galenus, or Galen, a Greek physician contributed much written material on early manual medicine

589 – 617 A.D. — Knowledge of massage and its applications were already well established in medicine at the time of the Sui Dynasty

1478 A.D. — *De Medicina* was rediscovered and became one of the first medical textbooks to be published using the newly invented Gutenberg printing press

1500 A.D.

1517 – 1590 — Ambrose Paré began to use massage techniques again for joint stiffness and wound healing after surgery

1776 – 1839 — Per Henrik Ling is given credit for the development of Swedish

1800 A.D.

1837 — M. LeRon brought the Movement Cure to Russia

1839 – 1909 — Dr. Johann Mezger of Holland is given credit for bringing massage to the scientific community

1852 – 1943 — John Harvey Kellogg, founder of the Battle Creek Sanitarium, wrote dozens of articles and two textbooks on massage and hydrotherapy

1856 — Charles Fayette Taylor and George Henry Taylor, two brothers, introduced the Swedish Movements to the United States

1879 — Douglas Graham writes a history of massage

1880 — Mary Putnam Jacobi and Victoria A. White, medical doctors and professors of medicine in New York City, research the benefits of massage and ice packs in the management of anemia

For use with Fritz: *Mosby's Fundamentals of Therapeutic Massage,* third edition.

Transparency Master 2 (cont'd)
Historical Timeline (Fig. 1-4)

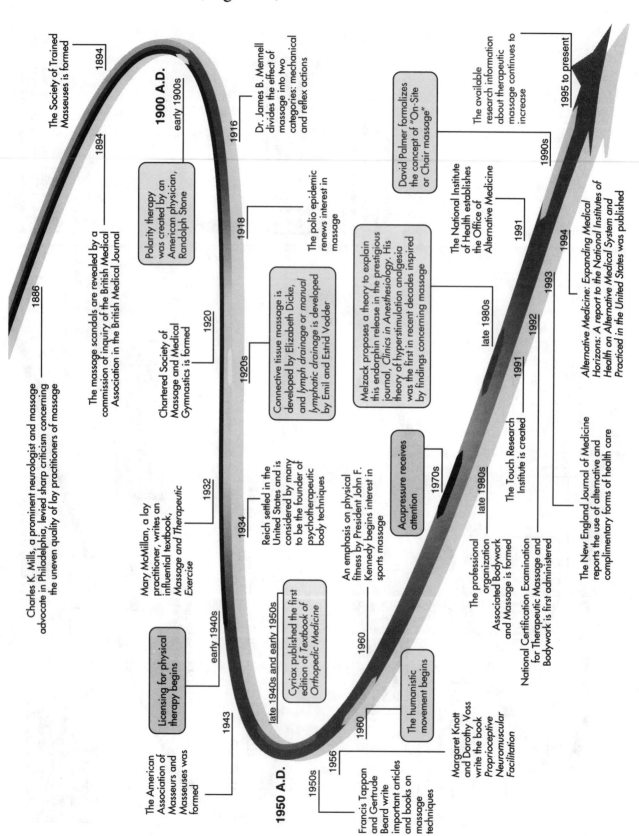

Normal Functions

Client displays resourceful functioning with good ability to respond to and recover from stress.

Massage Professional

Technician—500+ hours of education.

Health Care Supervision Required?

No.

Support Professionals

Fitness trainers, cosmetologists, wellness educators, prevention and healthy lifestyle focused health care and mental health professionals.

Dysfunctional and Complex Athletic Patterns

(Scope of practice encompasses Technician Level)

Client displays ability to function with effort and reduced ability to respond to and recover from stress. Recovery time is increased. Client demands extraordinary function of body.

Massage Professional

Practitioner—1000+ hours of education.

Illness/Trauma

(Scope of practice encompasses technician and practitioner levels)

Client displays function breakdown—substantially reduced ability to respond and recover or extensive healing period required such as with surgery and trauma.

Massage Professional

Therapist—2000+ hours of education.

Health Care or Athletic Trainer Supervision Required?

Possibly. No for wellness service and mild dysfunctional patterns. Moderate to identifiable dysfunctional pattern—Yes, but indirect; attention to referral needs is important.

Support Professionals

Athletic trainers—exercise physiologist, health care and mental health professionals—spiritually based support.

Health Care Supervision Required?

Yes. Direct supervision for all clients in this category; Possibly for dysfunctional category; No for wellness clients.

Support Professionals

Entire multidisciplinary team—health care/mental health professionals—spiritually based support.

■ Comprehensive scope of practice for therapeutic massage
☐ Wellness personal service scope of practice for therapeutic massage
▨ Dysfunctional and athletic patterns scope of practice for therapeutic massage
▨ Illness/trauma scope of practice for therapeutic massage

Transparency Master 4
Divisions of the Nervous System (Fig. 4-1)

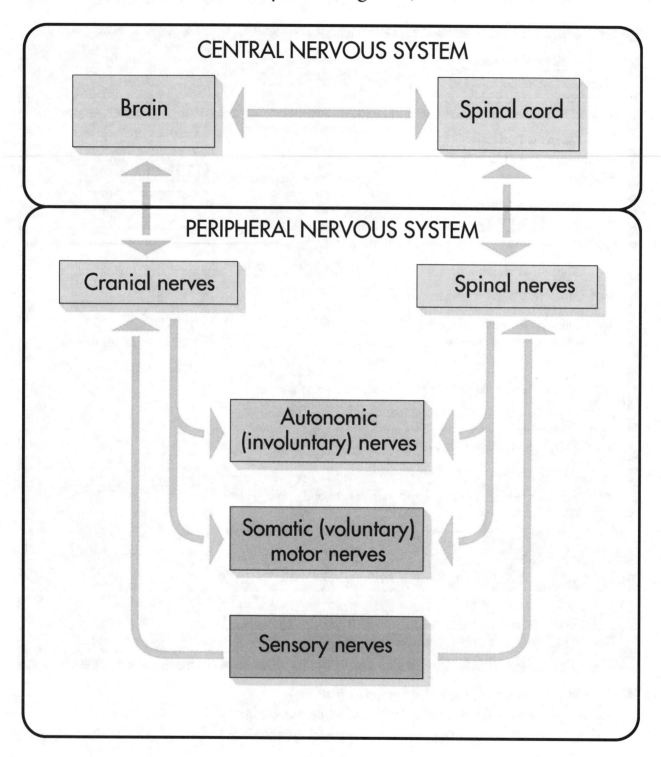

Transparency Master 5

Acupuncture Points, Motor Points, and Cutaneous Nerves (Fig. 4-2, *A*)

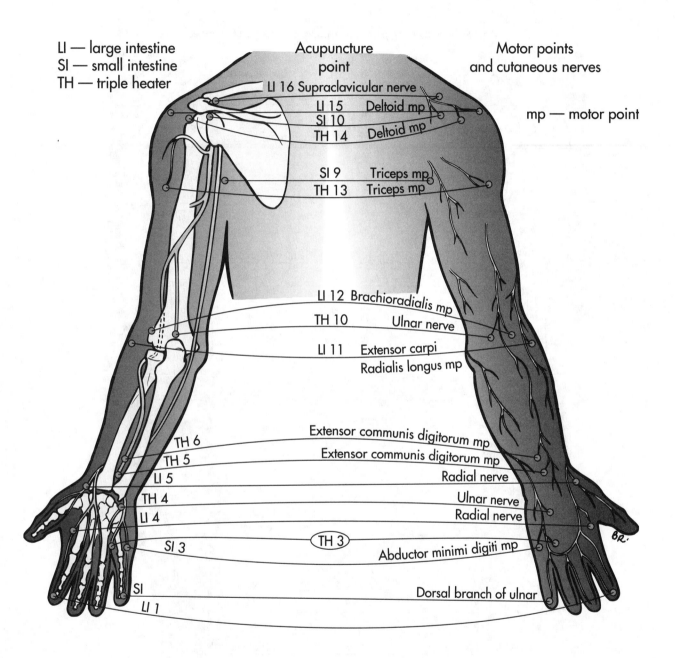

LI — large intestine
SI — small intestine
TH — triple heater

Acupuncture point

Motor points and cutaneous nerves

mp — motor point

LI 16 Supraclavicular nerve
LI 15 — Deltoid mp
SI 10
TH 14 — Deltoid mp

SI 9 — Triceps mp
TH 13 — Triceps mp

LI 12 Brachioradialis mp
TH 10 — Ulnar nerve
LI 11 — Extensor carpi
Radialis longus mp

TH 6
TH 5 — Extensor communis digitorum mp
LI 5 — Extensor communis digitorum mp
— Radial nerve
TH 4 — Ulnar nerve
LI 4 — Radial nerve
SI 3 — TH 3
— Abductor minimi digiti mp
SI — Dorsal branch of ulnar
LI 1

BR.

Continued

Transparency Master 5 (cont'd)
Acupuncture Points, Motor Points, and Cutaneous Nerves (Fig. 4-2, *B*)

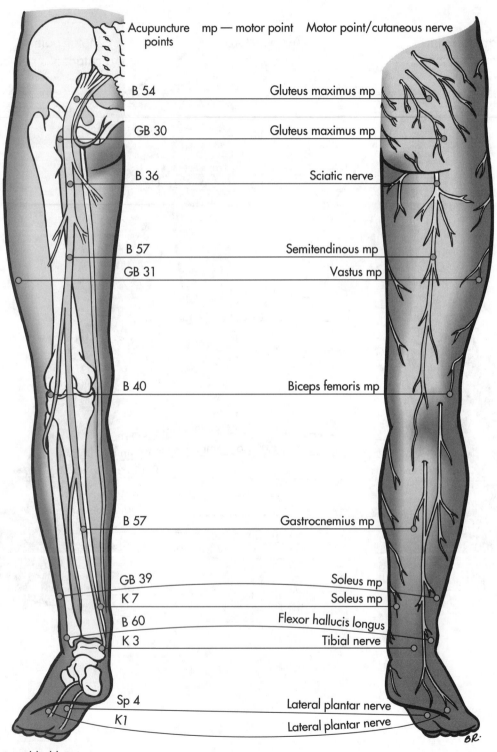

Acupuncture points   mp — motor point   Motor point/cutaneous nerve

Acupuncture point	Motor point/cutaneous nerve
B 54	Gluteus maximus mp
GB 30	Gluteus maximus mp
B 36	Sciatic nerve
B 57	Semitendinous mp
GB 31	Vastus mp
B 40	Biceps femoris mp
B 57	Gastrocnemius mp
GB 39	Soleus mp
K 7	Soleus mp
B 60	Flexor hallucis longus
K 3	Tibial nerve
Sp 4	Lateral plantar nerve
K 1	Lateral plantar nerve

B — bladder
GB — gallbladder
K — kidney
Sp — spleen

Transparency Master 6
Major Nerve Plexuses (Fig. 4-5)

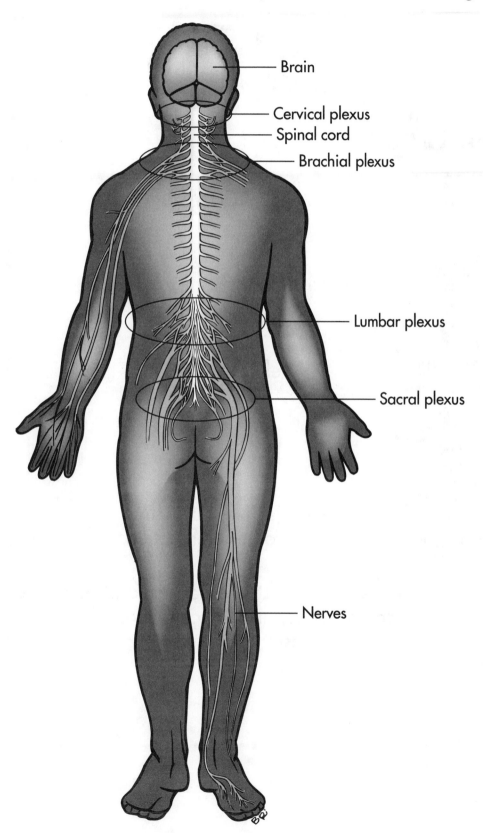

- Brain
- Cervical plexus
- Spinal cord
- Brachial plexus
- Lumbar plexus
- Sacral plexus
- Nerves

Transparency Master 7
Benefits of Massage (Unnumbered Fig. 5-1)

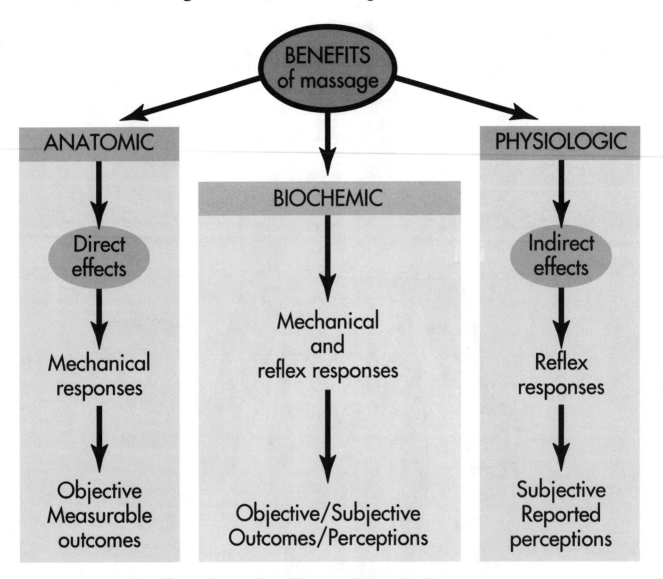

The benefits, effects, responses, and outcomes
can occur separately, combined, or as a
result of one another

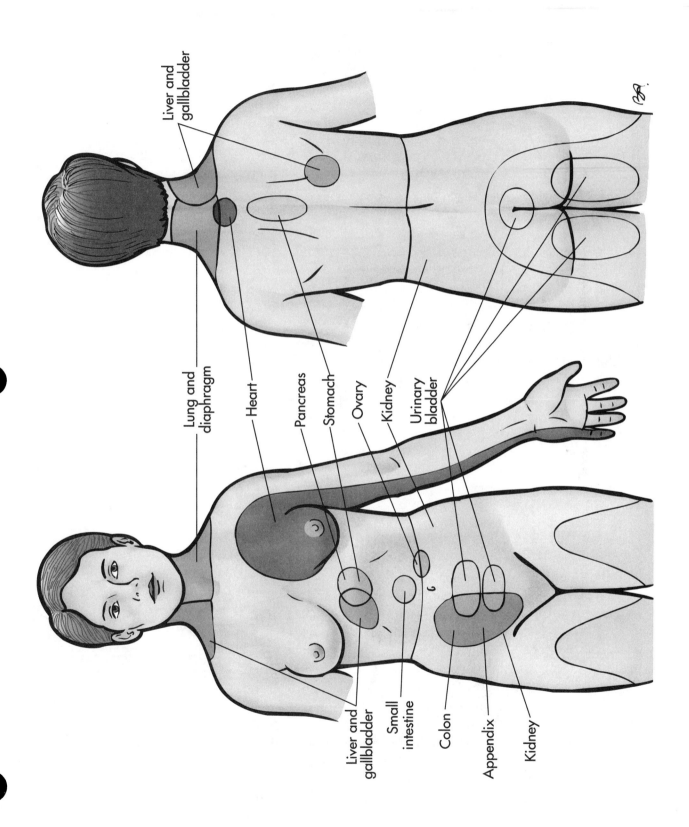

Liver and gallbladder

Lung and diaphragm

Heart

Pancreas

Stomach

Ovary

Kidney

Urinary bladder

Liver and gallbladder

Small intestine

Colon

Appendix

Kidney

Transparency Master 9

Endangerment Sites (Fig. 5-5, *A* and *B*)

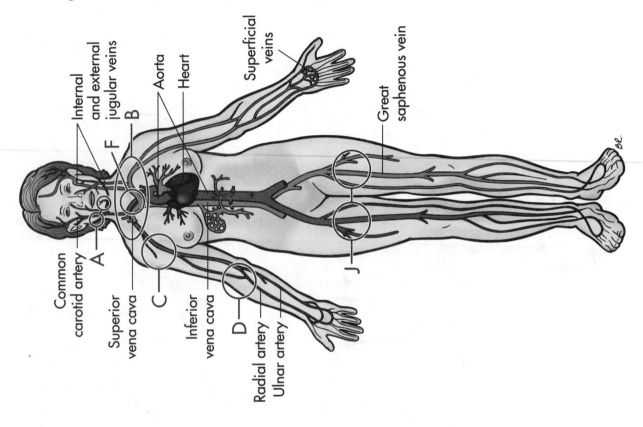

Internal and external jugular veins · Aorta · Heart · Superficial veins · Great saphenous vein · Common carotid artery · A · F · B · Superior vena cava · C · Inferior vena cava · D · Radial artery · Ulnar artery · J

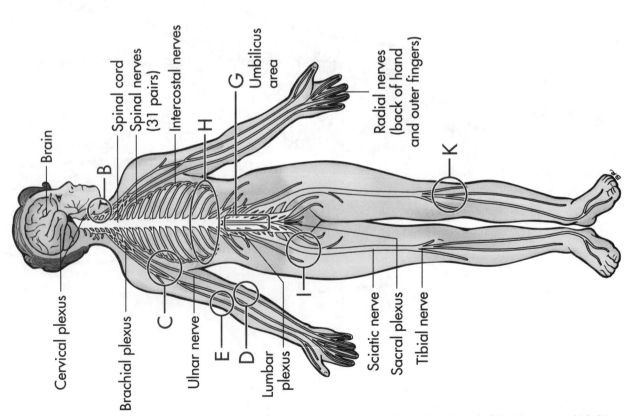

Brain · Spinal cord · Spinal nerves (31 pairs) · Intercostal nerves · Umbilicus area · Radial nerves (back of hand and outer fingers) · Cervical plexus · B · Brachial plexus · H · G · C · Ulnar nerve · E · D · Lumbar plexus · I · Sciatic nerve · Sacral plexus · Tibial nerve · K

Transparency Master 10
Body Mechanics for Compressive Force (Fig. 7-8)

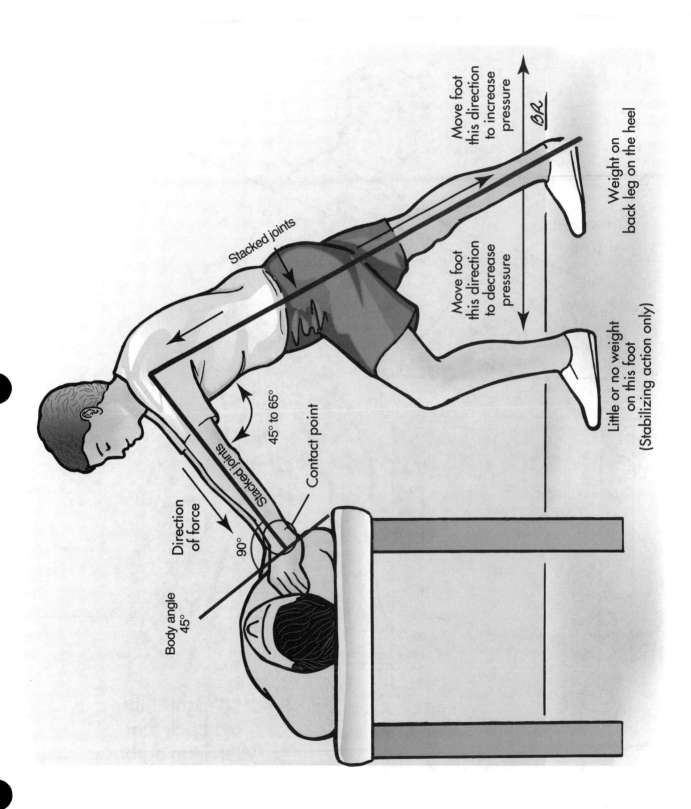

Move foot this direction to increase pressure

Move foot this direction to decrease pressure

Weight on back leg on the heel

Little or no weight on this foot (Stabilizing action only)

Stacked joints

45° to 65°

Contact point

Stacked joints

Direction of force

90°

Body angle 45°

Transparency Master 11
Body Mechanics for Petrissage and Stretching (Fig. 7-25)

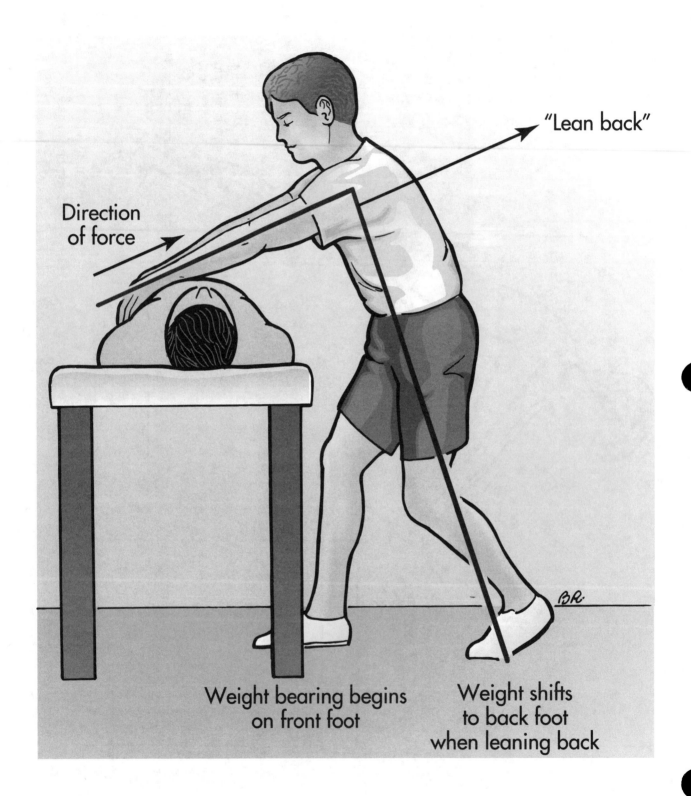

"Lean back"

Direction
of force

Weight bearing begins
on front foot

Weight shifts
to back foot
when leaning back

Transparency Master 12
Flow Pattern in the Colon (Fig. 9-5)

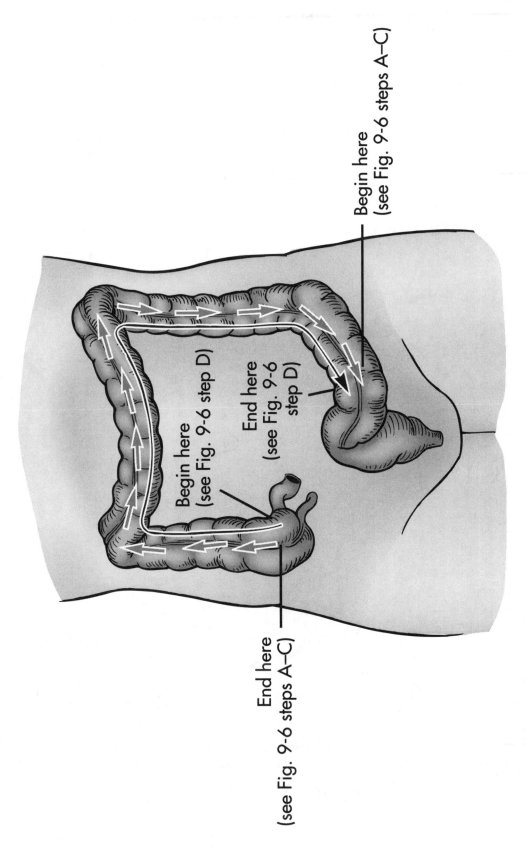

Begin here
(see Fig. 9-6 steps A–C)

Begin here
(see Fig. 9-6 step D)

End here
(see Fig. 9-6 step D)

End here
(see Fig. 9-6 steps A–C)

Transparency Master 13
Joint Movements (Fig. 9-31)

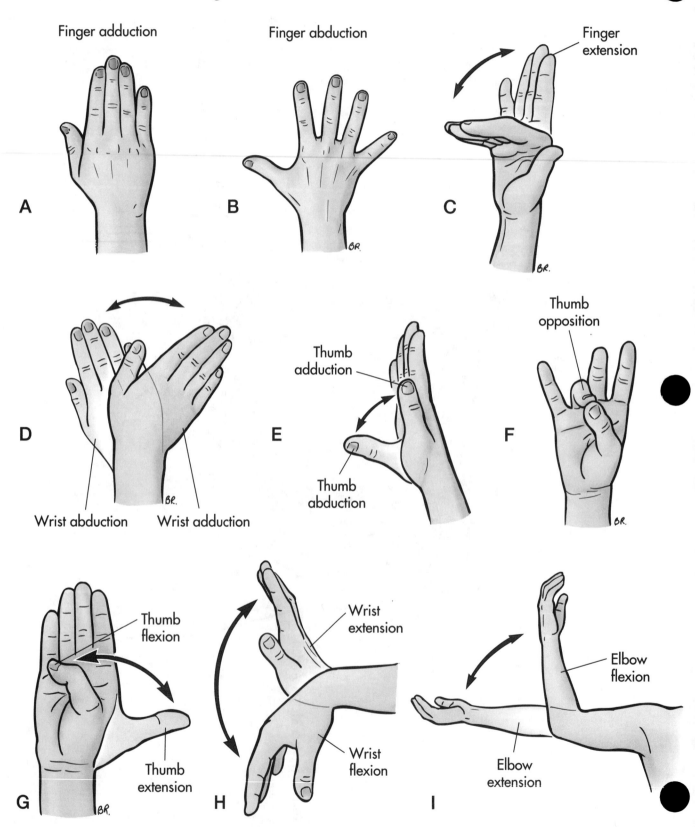

Finger adduction

Finger abduction

Finger extension

A

B

C

Wrist abduction   Wrist adduction

Thumb adduction

Thumb abduction

Thumb opposition

D

E

F

Thumb flexion

Thumb extension

Wrist extension

Wrist flexion

Elbow flexion

Elbow extension

G

H

I

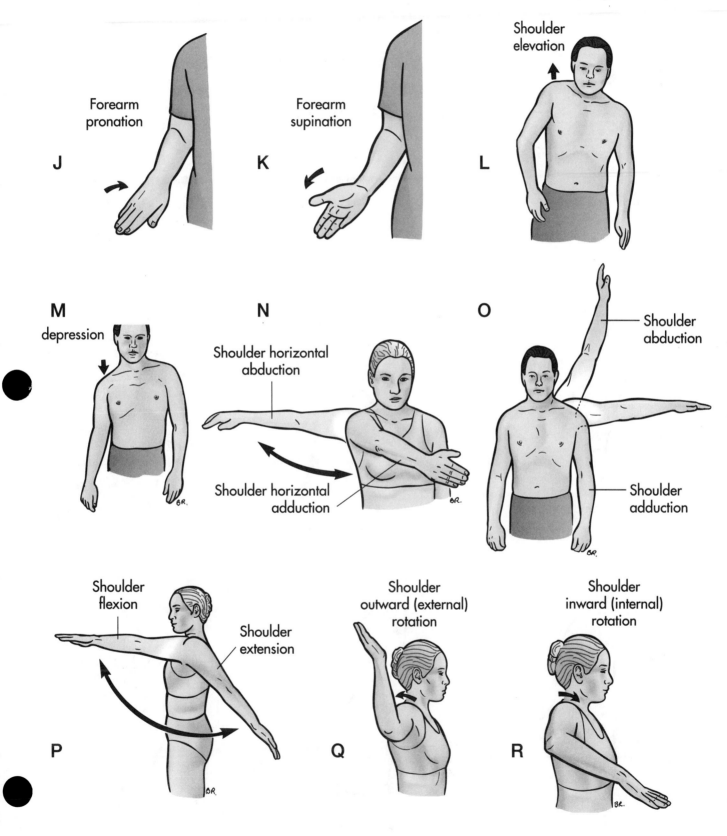

J Forearm pronation

K Forearm supination

L Shoulder elevation

M depression

N Shoulder horizontal abduction / Shoulder horizontal adduction

O Shoulder abduction / Shoulder adduction

P Shoulder flexion / Shoulder extension

Q Shoulder outward (external) rotation

R Shoulder inward (internal) rotation

Transparency Master 13 (cont'd)

Joint Movements (Fig. 9-31)

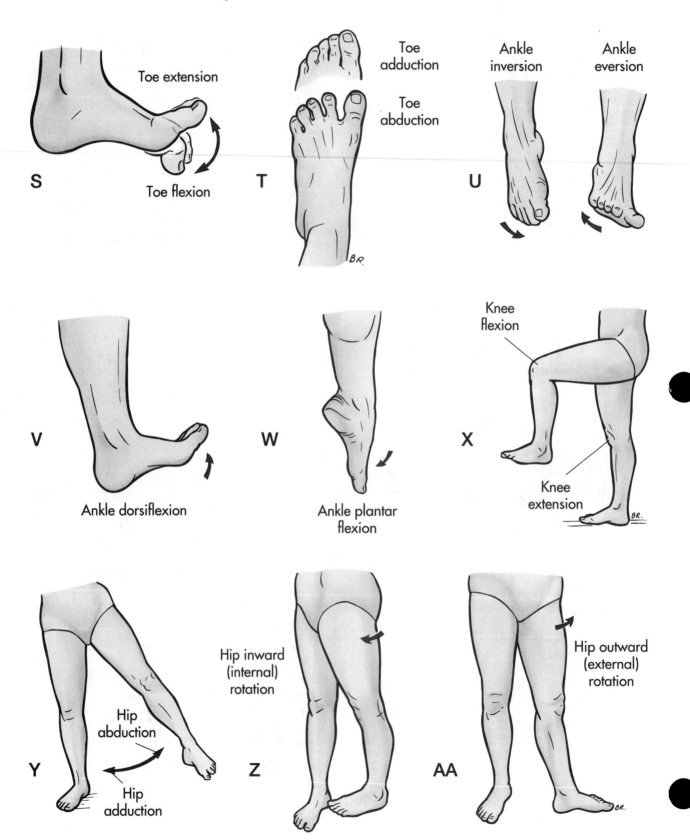

S — Toe extension / Toe flexion

T — Toe adduction / Toe abduction

U — Ankle inversion / Ankle eversion

V — Ankle dorsiflexion

W — Ankle plantar flexion

X — Knee flexion / Knee extension

Y — Hip abduction / Hip adduction

Z — Hip inward (internal) rotation

AA — Hip outward (external) rotation

For use with Fritz: *Mosby's Fundamentals of Therapeutic Massage*, third edition.

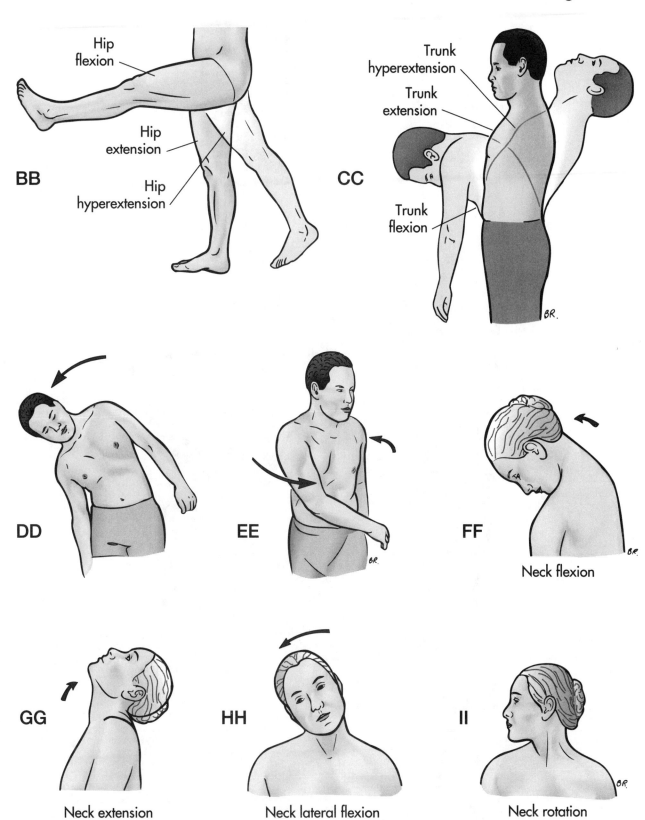

BB — Hip flexion, Hip extension, Hip hyperextension

CC — Trunk hyperextension, Trunk extension, Trunk flexion

DD

EE

FF — Neck flexion

GG — Neck extension

HH — Neck lateral flexion

II — Neck rotation

Transparency Master 14
Midline Balance Point (Fig. 10-2)

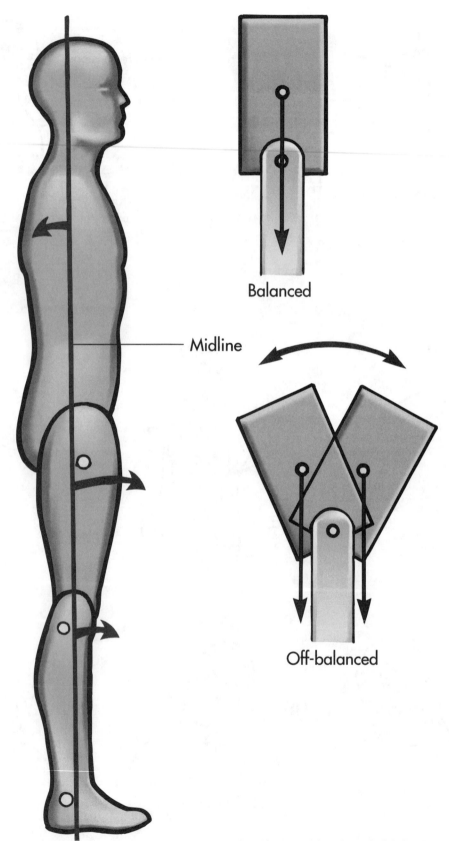

Balanced

Midline

Off-balanced

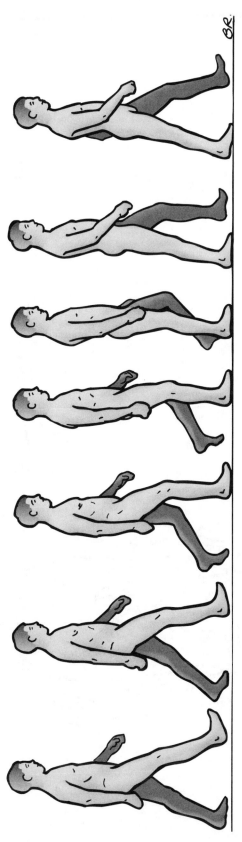

Transparency Master 16
Rocking Movement of the Sacral Iliac Joint (Fig. 10-7)

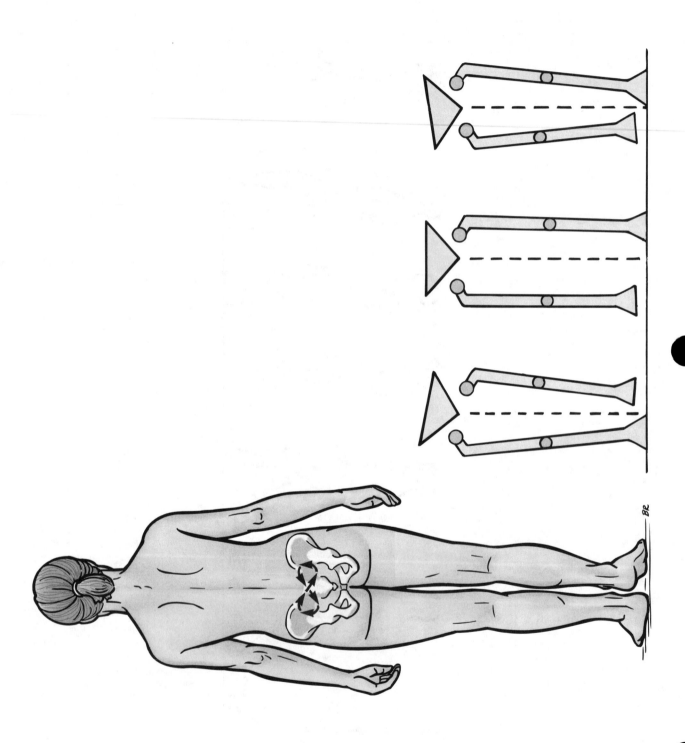

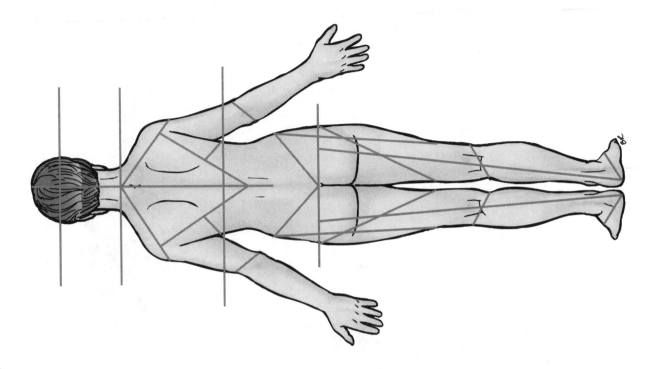

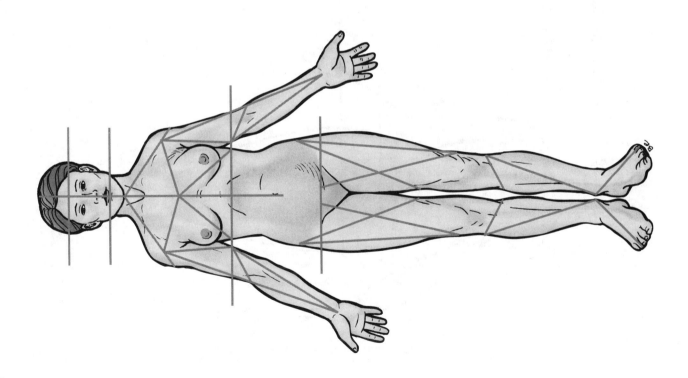

Transparency Master 18

Quadrants and Movement Segments (Fig. 10-16)

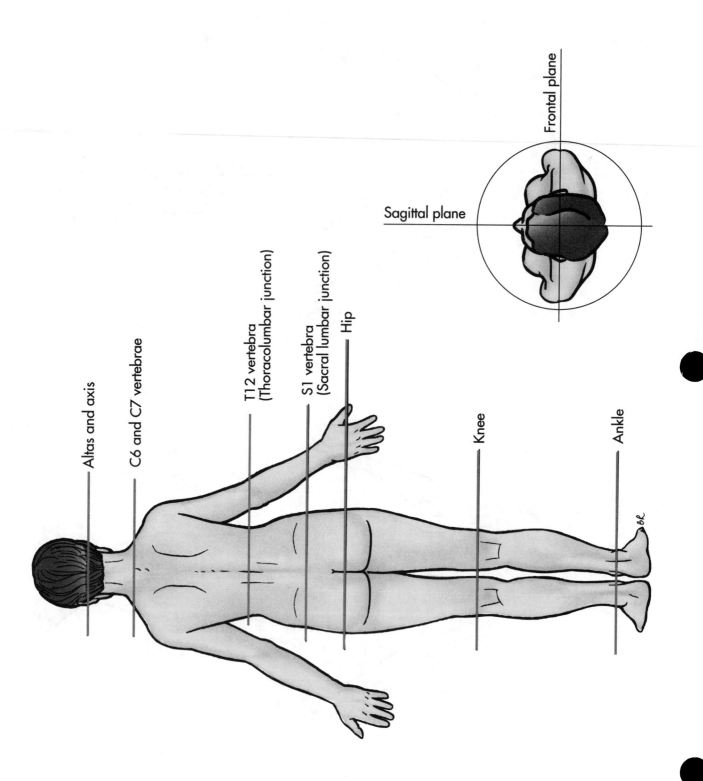

Transparency Master 19
Postural Influences on Muscle Patterns (Fig. 10-17)

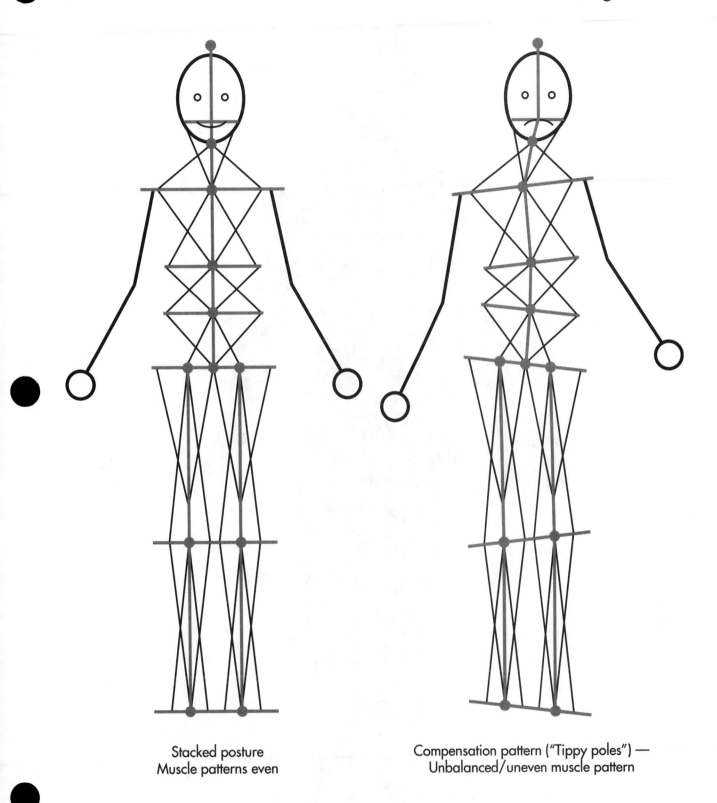

Stacked posture
Muscle patterns even

Compensation pattern ("Tippy poles") —
Unbalanced/uneven muscle pattern

Transparency Master 20
Strokes for Facilitating Lymphatic Flow (Fig. 11-8)

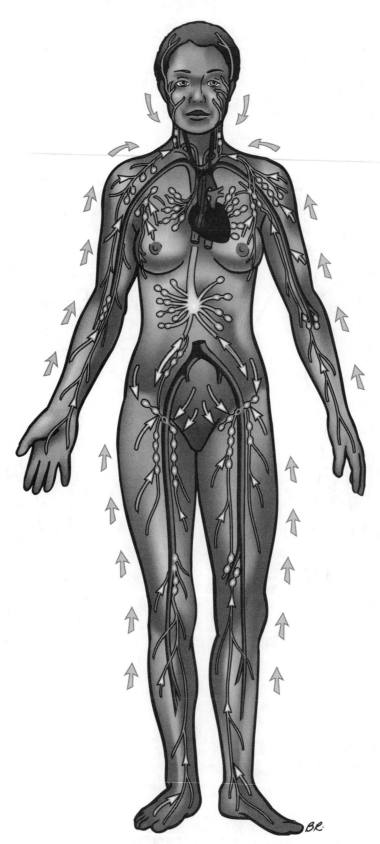

Transparency Master 21
Compression for Increasing Arterial Flow (Fig. 11-9)

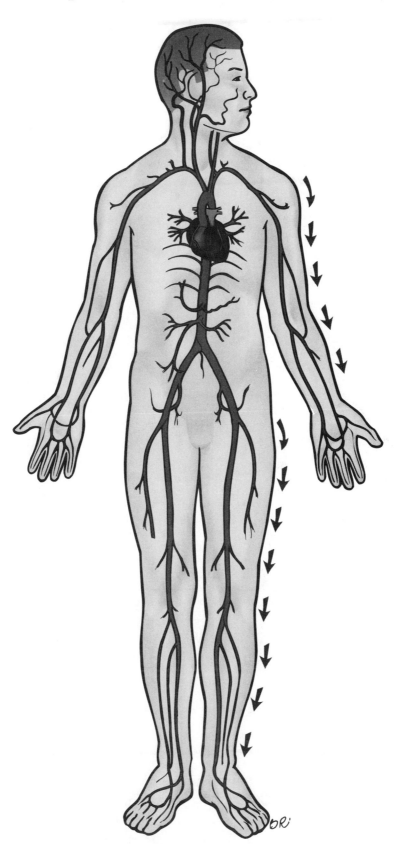

Transparency Master 22

Effleurage Strokes for Facilitating Venous Flow (Fig. 11-10)

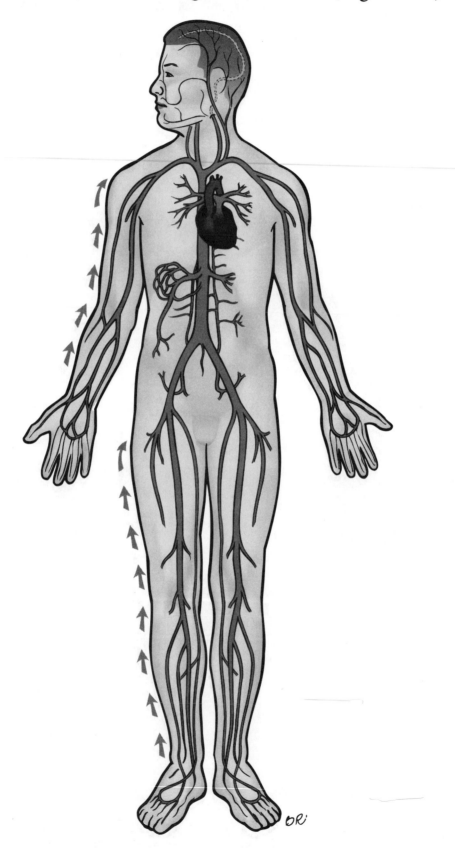

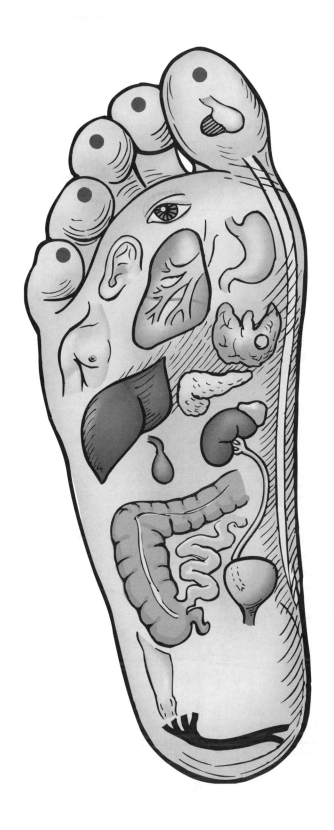
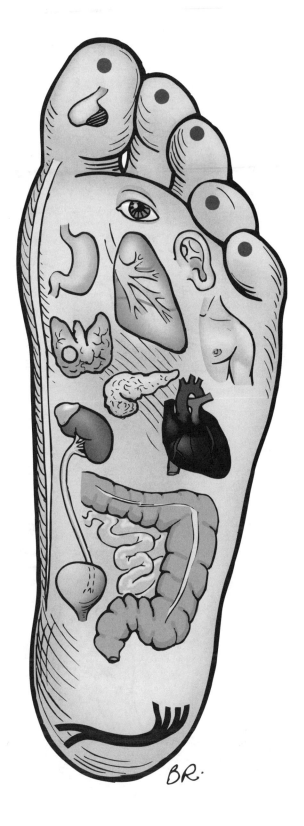

Transparency Master 24
Common Trigger Points (Fig. 11-15)

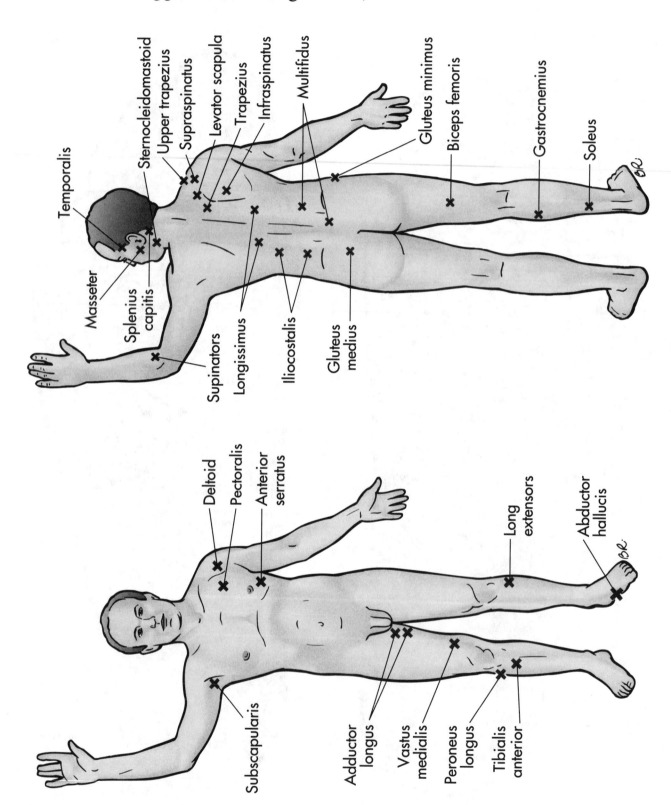

Transparency Master 25
Typical Locations of Meridians (Fig. 11-18)

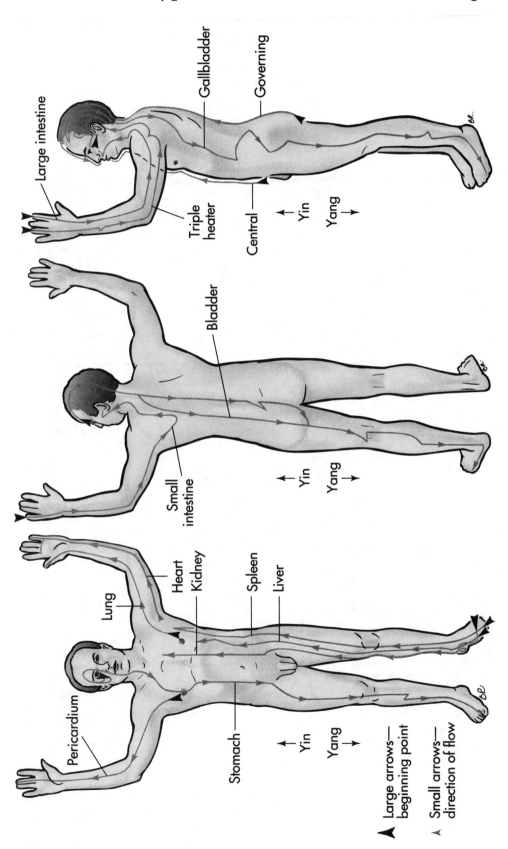

Gallbladder

Governing

Large intestine

Triple heater

Central

← Yin

Yang →

Bladder

Small intestine

← Yin

Yang →

Heart

Kidney

Lung

Spleen

Liver

Pericardium

Stomach

← Yin

Yang →

◄ Large arrows—beginning point

◄ Small arrows—direction of flow

Transparency Master 26

Relationship between the Five Elements and the Organs (Fig. 11-19)

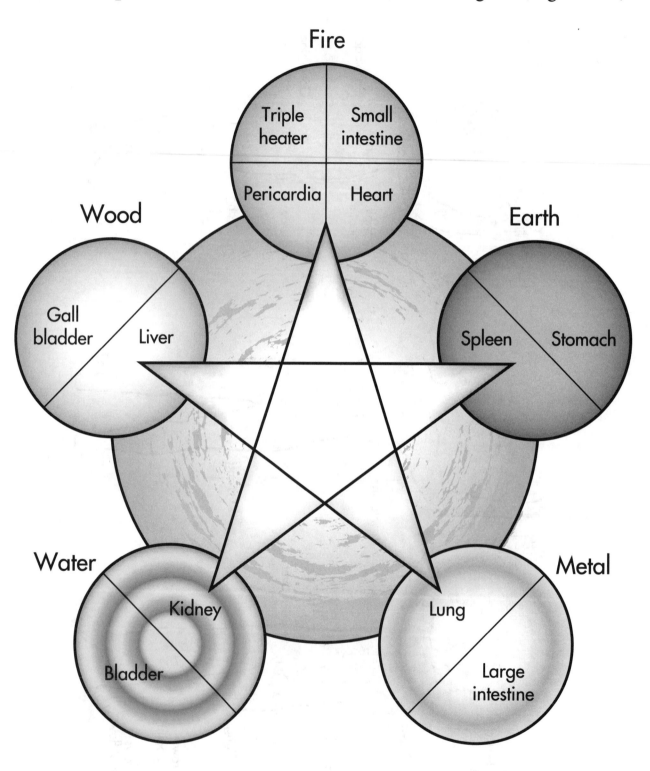

Fire

Triple heater | Small intestine
Pericardia | Heart

Wood

Gall bladder | Liver

Earth

Spleen | Stomach

Water

Kidney
Bladder

Metal

Lung
Large intestine

Transparency Master 27
Vertical Electromagnetic Currents (Fig. 11-22)

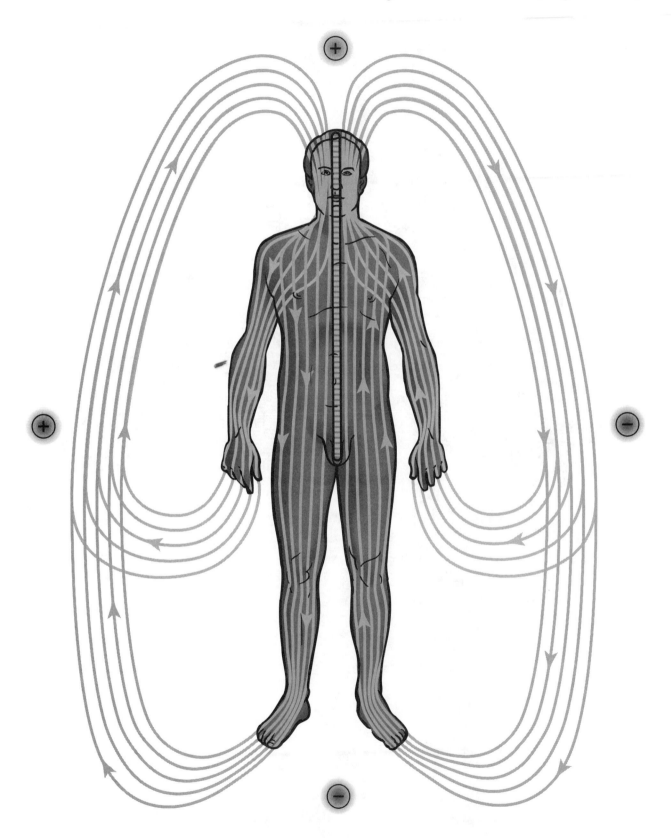

Transparency Master 28

Brain Wave Currents (Fig. 11-25)

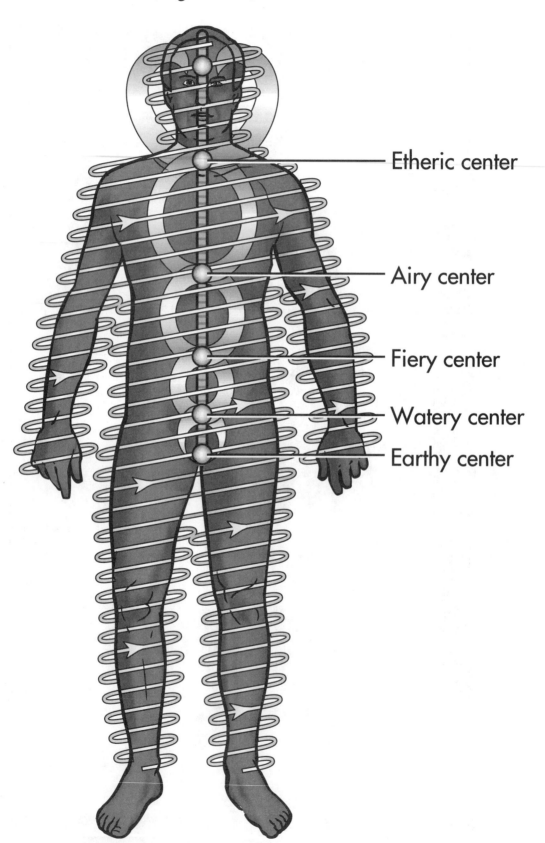

Etheric center

Airy center

Fiery center

Watery center

Earthy center

Transparency Master 29
Characteristics, Clinical Signs, and Interventions of Stages of Tissue Healing (Table 12-1)

Stages of Tissue Healing and Massage Interventions

	STAGE 1: ACUTE INFLAMMATORY REACTION	STAGE 2: SUBACUTE REPAIR AND HEALING	STAGE 3: CHRONIC MATURATION AND REMODELING
Characteristics	Vascular changes Inflammatory exudate Clot formation Phagocytosis, neutralization of irritants Early fibroblastic activity	Growth of capillary beds into area Collagen formation Granulation tissue; caution necessary Fragile, easily injured tissue	Maturation and remodeling of scar Contracture of scar tissue Collagen aligns along lines of stress forces (tensegrity)
Clinical Signs	Inflammation Pain prior to tissue resistance	Decreasing inflammation Pain during tissue resistance	Absence of inflammation Pain after tissue resistance
Massage Intervention	**Protection** Control and support effects of inflammation: PRICE Promote healing and prevent compensation patterns: Passive movement mid-range General massage and lymphatic drainage with caution. Support rest with full-body massage. 3 to 7 days	**Controlled Motion** Promote development of mobile scar Cautious and controlled soft tissue mobilization of scar tissue along fiber direction toward injury. Active and passive, open- and closed-chain range or motion, mid range. Support healing with full-body massage. 14 to 21 days	**Return to Function** Increase strength and alignment of scar tissue. Cross-fiber friction of scar tissue coupled with directional stroking along the lines of tension away from injury. Progressive stretching and active and resisted range of motion; full range. Support rehabilitation activities with full-body massage. 3 to 12 month